FREE Study Skills DVD Offer

Dear Customer,

Thank you for your purchase from Mometrix! We consider it an honor and privilege that you have purchased our product and want to ensure your satisfaction.

As a way of showing our appreciation and to help us better serve you, we have developed a Study Skills DVD that we would like to give you for <u>FREE</u>. **This DVD covers our "best practices" for studying for your exam, from using our study materials to preparing for the day of the test.**

All that we ask is that you email us your feedback that would describe your experience so far with our product. Good, bad or indifferent, we want to know what you think!

To get your **FREE Study Skills DVD**, email <u>freedvd@mometrix.com</u> with "FREE STUDY SKILLS DVD" in the subject line and the following information in the body of the email:

    a.   The name of the product you purchased.

    b.   Your product rating on a scale of 1-5, with 5 being the highest rating.

    c.   Your feedback. It can be long, short, or anything in-between, just your impressions and experience so far with our product. Good feedback might include how our study material met your needs and will highlight features of the product that you found helpful.

    d.   Your full name and shipping address where you would like us to send your free DVD.

If you have any questions or concerns, please don't hesitate to contact me directly.

Thanks again!

Sincerely,

Jay Willis
Vice President
<u>jay.willis@mometrix.com</u>
1-800-673-8175

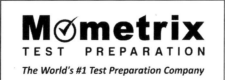

CNOR
Practice Questions

CNOR Practice Tests & Exam Review for the
CNOR Exam

Published by
Mometrix Test Preparation
CNOR Exam Secrets Test Prep Team

Written and edited by the CNOR Exam Secrets Test Prep Staff

Printed in the United States of America

This paper meets the requirements of ANSI/NISO Z39.48-1992 (Permanence of Paper).

Mometrix offers volume discount pricing to institutions. For more information or a price quote, please contact our sales department at sales@mometrix.com or 888-248-1219.

Mometrix Media LLC is not affiliated with or endorsed by any official testing organization. All organizational and test names are trademarks of their respective owners.

ISBN 13: 978-1-62120-044-4
ISBN 10: 1-62120-044-2

Table of Contents

Practice Test #1

Practice Questions

1. Identify the essential information required for the perioperative nurse assessment, performed in the Holding Area:
   a. Patient's exact age and weight
   b. Allergies, metal implants, and pacemakers
   c. Type and exact location of the surgery
   d. B and C

2. During a perioperative assessment, the O.R. nurse notices a red rash under the Ace bandage on the patient's wrist, and around his IV insertion site, which delivers normal saline solution. The patient complains the area is itchy and the nurse hears him wheezing. Identify the most likely problem:
   a. Possible latex allergy
   b. Bronchitis
   c. Hypersensitivity to IV solution
   d. Psychological fear of surgery

3. Choose the best method for confirming the exact surgical site with the patient during the perioperative assessment:
   a. Ask the patient to point to the surgical site, and then mark the area with a sticky note
   b. Ask the patient to show you where the surgery site will be, and then check if the surgeon marked it with a permanent marker
   c. If the patient cannot verbalize the surgical site, confirm the site with a family member or guardian, then mark the site with adhesive tape
   d. Check the surgical permit to confirm the proposed surgical site, then affirm correct marking

4. The person responsible for marking the surgical site is the:
   a. Patient
   b. Perioperative nurse
   c. Surgeon
   d. Anesthesiologist

5. Identify the responsibilities of the perioperative nurse:
   a. To assess the patient and develop the nursing diagnosis
   b. To identify desired outcomes and evaluate care
   c. To develop and execute a discharge plan
   d. A and B

6. Select the data that is NOT an essential component of the perioperative nurse assessment:
    a. Patient's diagnosis; current physical state; and psychosocial elements (literacy, language skills, important ethnic, cultural, spiritual or lifestyle data relevant to the surgery)
    b. Medical history; hospitalizations; previous surgeries; and major illnesses
    c. Verification of the patient's insurance coverage or ability to pay
    d. Patient's comprehension of the proposed procedure

7. Your patient is a surgical technologist, so as a safety precaution you must ask her:
    a. "What type of gloves do you use in the O.R.?"
    b. "Have you ever noticed a rash after removing latex gloves?"
    c. "Do you have an area of specialization in the OR?"
    d. A and B

8. Your breast biopsy patient is tearful during the perioperative nursing assessment, so her most likely nursing diagnosis is:
    a. Fear of body image change, pain or death
    b. Fear of medical personnel
    c. Fear of anaphylactic reaction
    d. Fear of missing work

9. To alleviate your patient's preoperative fear and anxiety, you must:
    a. Listen attentively
    b. Explain every detail of the proposed surgical procedure
    c. Provide reassurance
    d. A and C

10. Identify the psychosocial attribute important to your patient's comprehension of the procedure:
    a. Temperature, pulse and respiration
    b. Cultural beliefs regarding surgery
    c. Skin appearance
    d. Level of consciousness

11. When you diagnose your patient preoperatively with knowledge deficit and anxiety, your most important determination for the correct intervention is the:
    a. Etiology of the knowledge deficit
    b. Patient's education level
    c. Patient's coping ability
    d. Patient's cultural background

12. Choose the relevant factors for deep vein thrombosis (DVT), which you must identify when reviewing your patient's medical record:
    a. Age older than 50
    b. History of varicose veins
    c. History of ovarian cysts
    d. A and B

13. Sequential stockings (graduated compression stockings) dramatically reduce the incidence of:
   a. Pressure sores
   b. Infection
   c. Deep vein thrombosis (DVT)
   d. Electrical injury

14. The telephone interviewer obtained your patient's basic information preoperatively, but as the perioperative nurse, you must also:
   a. Go over each question again with your patient, then transport him to the O.R.
   b. Identify your patient, get a report from the Holding Area nurse, and review his Assessment sheet, including test results
   c. Review his laboratory findings, and then transport him to the O.R.
   d. Identify your patient, then transport him to the O.R.

15. Identify the areas of expertise essential for the perioperative nurse:
   a. Anatomy
   b. Surgical procedures, instruments and equipment
   c. Endotracheal tube insertion and internal physical landmarks
   d. A and B

16. Select the "never event" (the term coined in 2001 by Dr. Ken Kizer of the National Quality Forum to describe a surgical error):
   a. An appendix ruptures during surgery
   b. An Operating Room fire results in surgery on the wrong body part, patient death, or patient disability
   c. Simultaneous surgeries on multiple accident victims
   d. Hemorrhage after surgery on a cerebral aneurysm

17. Choose the most likely nursing diagnosis for a patient who experiences slightly elevated pulse, blood pressure, and respiratory rate while in the Holding Area:
   a. Hypertension
   b. COPD
   c. Anxiety
   d. Heart disease

18. Identify the methods for alleviating anxiety in the preoperative patient:
   a. Solicit questions related to the proposed surgical procedure
   b. Explain the surgical procedure and the post-operative expectations
   c. Have a set of practiced answers for all patients with specific surgeries
   d. A and B

19. ER staff notify you at 03:00 to prepare for three critical MVA patients; two of them require simultaneous multiple procedures. Identify the factors predisposing the surgical team to make wrong-site or wrong-patient errors:

    a. Emergency status, unusual time pressures, multiple surgeons, and simultaneous multiple procedures during a single session

    b. Emergency status, multiple vehicle accidents, and time pressure to prepare the operating theaters

    c. Unusual time pressures, multiple surgeons, and under-staffing

    d. Unusual time for surgery, multiple theaters, and pressure for on-call staff

20. Select the best methods to identify your preoperative patient at your first encounter, before beginning the assessment:

    a. Compare his wristband and chart, and ask him to spell his name

    b. Call his name and if he responds, compare his chart and wristband

    c. Check his chart, ask the patient to spell his name, and ask the Holding Area nurse to identify him

    d. Confirm the patient's identity with his relatives, check his wristband, and ask the Holding Area nurse to identify him

21. The purpose of a "time out" immediately before beginning a surgical procedure is to:

    a. Give the staff a break before beginning the surgery

    b. Verify the correct patient, procedure and site

    c. Confirm the availability of surgical implants, if applicable

    d. B and C

22. Identify the relevant information that the Holding Area nurse must relay to the O.R. Nurse:

    a. The patient has a grass allergy

    b. The patient's right leg is paralyzed

    c. The patient has a pacemaker implant

    d. B and C

23. "Hand-off" is complete when the Holding Area nurse communicates all relevant information to you, and then you:

    a. Introduce yourself to your patient, explain your role, identify him, and perform an assessment

    b. Observe your patient's status, and review with the Holding Area nurse any safety concerns, his background, and any actions taken or required

    c. Prioritize your actions (timing), identify all responsible parties (ownership), and determine what comes next

    d. A, B and C

24. Identify the three steps of the Universal Protocol for preventing wrong site, wrong procedure, and wrong person surgery:

    a. Preoperative verification; mark the operative site; and take a "time out" before starting surgery

    b. Assess allergies and implants; read the History for your patient's hospitalizations; and take a "time out" before taking your patient to the O.R.

    c. Mark the operative site; confirm the consent form was signed; and identify your patient

    d. Check the medication history; verify your patient's identity; confirm the operative site with the surgeon

25. When a sterilized laparotomy tray has a damp wrapper during prep, the O.R. Nurse must:
    a. Unwrap the tray to prevent its use, and send the entire contents back to CSS for resterilization
    b. Unwrap the tray, allow the scrub nurse to remove the instruments, and send only the tray back to CSS for resterilization
    c. Leave the tray wrapped until it dries, then it will be OK to use
    d. Open the tray on a ring stand and allow the scrub nurse use it from there

26. To ensure the patient remains free of infection, the Operating Room nurse must use:
    a. Excellent aseptic technique
    b. Proper preparation for the incision site
    c. Proper anesthesia
    d. A and B

27. Identify the proper tape for a sterile pack:
    a. Surgical adhesive tape
    b. Pressure-sensitive, striped chemical indicator tape
    c. Double-sided paper tape
    d. Extra-strength water resistant tape

28. The standard criterion for sterile packaging material is that it must:
    a. Resist tears, punctures, and abrasions
    b. Prevent infiltration and egress of sterilant
    c. Be waterproof
    d. Be puncture-proof

29. Identify the disadvantage of using rigid containers to hold sterile instruments:
    a. Weight
    b. Instrument damage
    c. Residual condensation
    d. A and C

30. Identify the exogenous sources of infection:
    a. Cracks in nail polish, artificial nails, and jewelry
    b. Talking, coughing, and breathing
    c. The patient's skin flora
    d. A and B

31. The position of the Joint Commission Association of periOperative Nurses (AORN), the Centers for Disease Control and Prevention (CDC), and the World Health Organization (WHO) regarding artificial nails worn by perioperative staff is that:
    a. Artificial nails present no registered concerns
    b. Properly maintained artificial nails harbor fewer microorganisms than natural nails
    c. Artificial nails must not be worn in the O.R.
    d. Artificial nails are safe when worn under double gloves

32. Identify the cause of the majority of surgical site infections (SSI):
    a. Poor aseptic technique
    b. The patient's own flora
    c. Respiratory contaminants from perioperative personnel
    d. Improperly cleaned lights in the operating theater

33. Identify the main modes of transmission for microorganisms in the O.R.:
    a. Droplet, airborne, and contact
    b. Body fluids, purulent material, and blood
    c. Sneezing, coughing, and talking
    d. Blood and dirty equipment

34. Choose the best definition of Universal Precautions, as required by the Center for Disease Control (CDC) since 1987?
    a. Universal Precautions are only necessary when caring for a patient with HIV/AIDS or hepatitis B
    b. Universal Precautions are necessary when the caregiver is exposed to any blood, semen, or vaginal secretions
    c. Universal Precautions are necessary when the caregiver is exposed to the patient's mucous membranes, blood, secretions, or excretions, except sweat
    d. Universal Precautions are necessary for all patients to prevent the transfer of any blood-borne pathogen, including human immunodeficiency virus (HIV), and hepatitis B (HBV)

35. Select the example of Universal Precautions standards:
    a. Use proper hand washing technique and carefully dispose of all sharps (blades, needles, and pointed instruments)
    b. Use proper PPE, such as gloves, masks, and gowns
    c. Recap or remove all needles to prevent accidental punctures
    d. A and B

36. Identify the purpose of aseptic practice:
    a. To sterilize the skin by eliminating all bacteria
    b. To prevent contamination of an open wound with infectious agents
    c. To maintain a sterile field isolated from the adjacent unsterilized area
    d. B and C

37. The most important piece of protective equipment used by O.R. personnel during a bronchoscopy is a:
    a. Gown
    b. Mask with shield and goggles
    c. Gloves
    d. Shoe covers

38. Choose the correct steps to prep a laceration extending through your patient's eyebrow for suturing:
    a. Shave his eyebrow
    b. Irrigate his wound with prep solution, taking care to avoid splashing solution into his eye
    c. Apply ophthalmic ointment into his eye to protect it
    d. A and C

39. Identify how the length of surgical prep time is determined:
    a. The O.R. Committee sets the prep time
    b. Researchers who studied the effectiveness of the antimicrobial agents set the prep time
    c. The manufacturer's recommendations set the prep time
    d. B and C

40. Select the best instruction to give a student nurse who placed the sterile drape on the operative area, when you notice it slid down several inches.
    a. "Reposition the drape over the incision site and continue draping."
    b. "Discard that drape and ask the circulating nurse for a new one."
    c. "Remove the contaminated drape and place it on the back table."
    d. "Tell the circulating nurse to re-prep the surgical area, and then drape it again with sterile material."

41. You observe a newly hired perioperative nurse remove his mask and pocket it for use in the next procedure, to save money. Choose your best response to his action:
    a. "Thanks for cost-saving. Just allow your mask to hang around your neck between procedures. Please don't put it in your pocket."
    b. "Bag your used mask before you put it in your pocket. If you reuse your mask for cost-saving, don't contaminate it."
    c. "Your mask is contaminated by microorganisms from your respiratory tract and from the procedure. Discard your mask after each procedure. Thanks for your concern, but safety surpasses saving money."
    d. "Masks are expensive and your concern over cost-saving is admirable."

42. Choose the TRUE statement regarding ethylene oxide gas:
    a. Ethylene oxide is toxic, explosive and flammable
    b. Ethylene oxide sterilizes items that cannot tolerate moist heat or steam sterilization, like plastic or rubber
    c. Ethylene oxide is nontoxic
    d. A and B

43. You drop a unique instrument needed to complete the surgery in progress. Choose the best response by the circulating nurse:
    a. Don gloves; retrieve the instrument; sanitize it; flash sterilize it; return it to the scrub nurse
    b. Call area hospitals; borrow a similar instrument that is sterile; re-schedule the surgery
    c. Retrieve the instrument with a sterile towel; send it to Central Sterile Supply for processing; return it to the scrub nurse
    d. Don gloves; retrieve the instrument; soak it in alcohol for 5 minutes; return it to the scrub nurse

44. Identify the necessary precaution the nurse takes when placing a patient in the lithotomy position, to prevent patient injury during the surgery:
    a. Lift the patient's legs slowly
    b. Lift only one of the patient's legs at time
    c. Lift both of the patient's legs in unison
    d. A and C

45. Choose the correct rule for performing a surgical prep:
    a. Start cleaning at the dirtiest area first to allow the prep solution time to kill the bacteria
    b. Start cleaning at the incision area first, then prep in circles radiating outward
    c. Start cleaning at the patient's midline, then prep outward toward the extremities
    d. None of the above

46. Choose the TRUE statement regarding the table strap:
    a. Apply the table strap after the patient is asleep
    b. Position the table strap 2 inches above the patient's knees
    c. Position the table strap 2 inches below the patient's knees
    d. Remove the table strap as soon as the patient is extubated

47. Indicate the necessary precaution the nurse must take when lowering the patient's legs from the lithotomy position:
    a. Extend the patient's legs completely, to prevent hip abduction
    b. Lower the patient's legs quickly, to reduce back strain
    c. Lower the patient's legs slowly, to prevent severe hypotension
    d. A and C

48. Identify the major concern regarding jackknife positioning:
    a. Venous pooling in the feet and chest
    b. Restricted diaphragm movement, which decreases cardiac output and ventilation
    c. Increased risk of injury to the eye and ear
    d. A and B

49. A metal implant in your patient's right hip means you must place the dispersive electrode:
    a. To avoid putting the metal implant in the circuit path
    b. On an extra large dispersive electrode pad
    c. On his right thigh
    d. A and B

50. Choose the proper procedure for attaching a blade to a scalpel handle:
    a. Grasp the blade firmly between your index finger and thumb, then attach the blade to the handle
    b. Use a needle holder to attach the blade to the handle
    c. Open the blade package, but leave its sharp end covered while you attach its blunt end to the handle, then remove the package completely
    d. Grasp the blade with toothed forceps and attach it to the handle

51. Identify the FALSE statement regarding an ultrasonic scalpel:
    a. An ultrasonic scalpel vibrates 55,000 times per second
    b. Increasing power to the ultrasonic scalpel boosts its cutting and coagulating ability
    c. An ultrasonic scalpel cuts and coagulates simultaneously
    d. An ultrasonic scalpel denatures protein to create a sticky coagulant

52. Identify the TRUE statement regarding an Army-Navy retractor:
    a. An Army-Navy retractor is self-retaining
    b. An Army-Navy retractor is like a Balfour with a blade
    c. An Army-Navy retractor is double-ended
    d. An Army-Navy retractor contains a suction port

53. Identify the nonabsorbable suture:
    a. Mersilene (polyester)
    b. Chromic gut
    c. Vicryl
    d. Plain surgical gut

54. The best definition of "surgical gut" is a:
    a. Type of nonabsorbable suture
    b. Suture made from the intestines of a cat
    c. Suture derived from the collagen of the submucosal layer of sheep, cattle or hog intestines
    d. Suture made from nylon

55. Choose the TRUE statement regarding silk sutures:
    a. Silk sutures are thread from silkworm larvae cocoons
    b. Silk suture strands are twisted or braided
    c. Silk sutures never absorb into the patient's body
    d. A and B

56. Choose the TRUE statement regarding blunt-tip surgical needles:
    a. The surgeon's assistant uses a blunt-tip needle for skin closure
    b. Blunt-tip needles are available in several gauges
    c. Blunt-tip needles are for internal suturing
    d. B and C

57. Choose the TRUE statement regarding skin staples:
    a. Press the stapler firmly against the incision line
    b. "Kiss" the skin gently with the stapler when applying skin staples
    c. Place the staples ½ inch apart
    d. A and C

58. Choose the best explanation that accounts for shearing injuries while moving an anesthetized patient:
    a. Shearing occurs when the patient's skin remains stationary and the tissue beneath it shifts
    b. Shearing occurs when perioperative personnel pull a patient, rather than lift him
    c. Shearing occurs when the nurse inadequately pads the patient's bony prominences
    d. A and B

59. You position your Mayo stand over the patient and prepare to pass instruments to the surgeon. The surgeon, who is very tall, instructs the anesthetist to raise the operating table. Choose your most appropriate action:
    a. Request a step stool, so you can view the surgical field clearly
    b. Move your Mayo stand to the foot of the operating table
    c. Raise your Mayo stand to avoid injuring the patient
    d. A and C

60. Select the conditions most likely to increase your patient's risk of pressure ulcers:
    a. Diabetes and vascular disease
    b. Heart disease and arthritis
    c. Chronic kidney stone formation and gout
    d. Ulcerative colitis and chronic kidney disease

61. Identify the nurse's main safety concern during facial surgery:
    a. Use 100% oxygen (O2)
    b. Drape the patient to prevent pockets of oxygen (O2) from accumulating
    c. Coat the patient's facial hair with water-soluble lubricant
    d. B and C

62. Select the TRUE statement regarding thrombin for hemostasis:
    a. Thrombin is derived from porcine pancreas and controls capillary bleeding
    b. Mix thrombin just prior to use because it loses potency after 20 minutes
    c. Thrombin a dry white powder, reconstituted with saline or water, and combined with oxidized cellulose
    d. Bovine-derived thrombin can trigger an autoimmune response, resulting in a hemorrhage

63. Select the TRUE statement regarding lasers:
    a. Carbon dioxide (CO2) lasers cannot damage the cornea
    b. Argon lasers can damage the cornea
    c. Neodymium-Yttrium-Aluminum-Garnet (Nd:YAG) lasers can damage the retina
    d. Optical damage occurs with carbon dioxide (CO2) lasers only

64. Identify the nurse's safety precaution before the surgeon uses a laser:
    a. Ensure everyone in the room wears appropriate eye protection, even for endoscopic laser procedures
    b. Place a "DANGER, Laser Radiation" sign at every Procedure Room entrance or exit
    c. Do not cover the window in the O.R. door or any other windows, since laser beams do not penetrate glass
    d. A and B

65. Identify the usual incision for an appendectomy:
    a. Midline
    b. McBurney
    c. Midabdominal transverse
    d. Thoracoabdominal

66. Select the synonym meaning "suprapubic incision":
    a. Midabdominal transverse incision
    b. Subcostal incision
    c. Pfannenstiel incision
    d. Lower oblique inguinal incision

67. Identify the two structures the surgeon joins to form the anastomosis during a complete gastrectomy:
    a. Esophagus and jejunum
    b. Jejunum and colon
    c. Esophagus and duodenum
    d. Esophagus and colon

68. Identify the major advantage of laparoscopic surgery:
    a. A reduced infection risk for the patient
    b. The surgeon's increased capacity to inspect the patient's abdomen
    c. The patient's reduced potential for DVT
    d. The patient's decreased venous return

69. Identify the equipment the nurse must count at the close of surgery:
    a. Kitner dissectors, lap sponges (pads), 4" x 4" RAY-TEC® (x-ray detectable) sponges
    b. Gauze peanuts, tonsil sponges, cottonoid patties (neuro sponges)
    c. Thrombin-soaked gelatin sponges
    d. A and B

70. Choose the TRUE statement regarding formaldehyde as a specimen preservative:
    a. The nurse does not require gloves if the formaldehyde is diluted with water
    b. Formaldehyde is a proven carcinogen, so the nurse always requires gloves and proper ventilation
    c. The only requirement is for the nurse to decant the formaldehyde slowly
    d. The nurse must wear goggles, gloves, and a respirator when pouring formaldehyde

71. Identify the precaution the perioperative nurse takes to avoid plume formation (smoke) during electrosurgery:
    a. Suction with an in-line filter to evacuate smoke
    b. Leave O.R. doors open to vent smoke into the hallway
    c. Wear a laser mask to avoid inhaling the smoke plume
    d. A and C

72. Choose the correct definition for a clean contaminated surgical wound:
    a. An incision that does not pierce the GI, respiratory, or GU tracts
    b. An incision that pierces the GI, respiratory, or GU tracts by controlled means
    c. A surgical site that contains infected or dead tissue
    d. An incision that is grossly contaminated, but with no sign of infection

73. You don a sterile gown and gloves, using the open glove technique. Your scrubbed thumb touches the outside of your second sterile glove. Choose your most appropriate next step:
    a. Continue gloving; your hand is bacteria-free, so you are uncontaminated
    b. Discard your contaminated gloves and ask for new ones
    c. Remove both your gown and gloves, then return to the scrub sink to start over
    d. Continue gloving, and then rinse your hands in sterile saline

74. You scrub according to hospital protocol, then accidentally touch the faucet with your hand while rinsing. Choose your most appropriate next step:
    a. Proceed into the O.R.
    b. Rinse for an extra minute, and then proceed to the O.R.
    c. Start your scrub over from the beginning, using a new scrub sponge/brush
    d. Wear double gloves on your contaminated hand, and proceed to the O.R.

75. You wear a sterile gown and gloves. The surgeon asks you to come to the opposite side of the O.R. table. Choose the most appropriate way to pass by other gowned and gloved staff:
    a. Front-to-front
    b. Your back to the operating table, and your front to the other staffer
    c. Back-to-back
    d. Side-to-side

76. You prepare for a scheduled surgery by opening the sterile packs and instruments. The scrub nurse sets up. The float nurse informs you there will be a two-hour delay. Choose your best response:
    a. Cover the sterile tables before you and the scrub nurse go to lunch
    b. Take turns with the scrub nurse to constantly monitor the sterile fields
    c. Discard the sterile set-up and order a new one from CSS
    d. Leave the O.R. doors open, so the float nurse can check the sterile fields when passing, and offer to help in another room

77. Identify the retractors:
    a. Richardson, Army-Navy, and Deaver
    b. Allis, Babcock, and Kocher
    c. Towel clip and sponge forceps
    d. Castroviejo, Metzenbaum, and Mayo

78. Name the color of an air line on an anesthesia machine:
    a. Green
    b. Yellow
    c. Blue
    d. White

79. Define suture "memory" and indicate how to eliminate it:
    a. "Memory" means the suture material returns to its original configuration; gently stretch it without applying tension to its swaged section
    b. "Memory" refers to a suture material made from metal; bend it until it is straight
    c. "Memory" refers to a suture that knots easily; dip it in water prior to passing it to the surgeon
    d. "Memory" refers to a suture that has to be loaded onto a needle; load several needle holders at once

80. Choose the best precaution before wrapping an Esmarch bandage around your patient's arm.
    a. Lower the arm to allow for venous stasis
    b. Raise the arm to allow for venous drainage
    c. Scrub the arm with povidone prep solution (Betadine)
    d. Shave and then scrub the arm with povidone prep solution (Betadine)

81. You 'scrub-in' on an emergency case. In the rush to set up, the circulating nurse opens sterile 3" x 3" sponges onto your back table. Choose your best response:
    a. Count the 3" x 3" sponges and keep them as/is on your back table
    b. Count the 3" x 3" sponges and use them to control hemorrhaging
    c. Discard the 3" x 3" sponges, so they will not be confused with radiopaque 4" x 4" sponges
    d. Count the 3" x 3" sponges and use them on sponge sticks

82. The scrub nurse discards soiled sponges into the kick-buckets. Identify the acceptable technique for the circulating nurse to handle and count soiled sponges:
   a. If the sponge has a clean end, the circulator does not need gloves to grasp it. The circulator places 5 or 10 sponges in each plastic bag.
   b. The circulator wears gloves, or uses a sponge stick to handle all sponges. The circulator counts sponges with the scrub nurse. When 5 or 10 accumulate, the circulator places them in a plastic bag and ties it closed.
   c. The circulator lines up all soiled sponges across an impervious pad on the floor, so all sponges are clearly visible for the final count.
   d. The circulator wears gloves or uses a sponge stick to place all soiled sponges in bags of 5 or 10. The circulator only performs the final count with scrub nurse.

83. Select the FALSE statement regarding pulse oximetry:
   a. Readings under 90% indicate significant hypoxemia
   b. Bright lights can interfere with the pulse oximeter's accuracy
   c. Methylene blue and other intravenous dyes diminish the pulse oximeter's accuracy
   d. Pulse oximetry measures oxygenation and ventilation

84. You are the circulating nurse. The anesthesiologist asks you to perform the Sellick maneuver, which means you must:
   a. Hold your patient's hand during induction
   b. Open the endotracheal tube and hand it to the anesthesiologist
   c. Press on your patient's cricoid cartilage
   d. Lift your patient's shoulders

85. Identify the most likely injury to result from faulty positioning that impairs blood-flow to the patient's legs:
   a. Phlebothrombosis
   b. Shearing
   c. Air embolism
   d. Bronchial spasm

86. Identify the body part that, if incorrectly positioned, results in brachial plexus injury:
   a. Leg
   b. Back
   c. Arm
   d. Head

87. Select the additional responsibility of a registered nurse while monitoring a moderately sedated patient, or one who received analgesia:
   a. The monitoring nurse should have no other responsibility that would distract from the monitors or from the patient
   b. Circulating, providing the nurse can see all the monitors
   c. The monitoring nurse can scrub in, providing all the monitors are visible from the field
   d. The monitoring nurse records the surgery, to help the circulating nurse

88. Identify the gastrointestinal organ that contains the cardia, fundus, corpus, and pylorus:
    a. Gall bladder
    b. Pancreas
    c. Stomach
    d. Small intestine

89. Identify the functions of the stomach:
    a. Acceptance and storage of ingested substances
    b. Digestion through gastric lipase, pepsinogen, and hydrochloric acid
    c. Absorption of essential nutrients with 95% efficiency
    d. A and B

90. Choose the synonym for 'bariatric surgery':
    a. Gall bladder surgery
    b. Weight reduction surgery
    c. Surgery on the elderly
    d. Surgery on the pancreas

91. Identify the procedure for direct visualization of the biliary tract:
    a. ERCP
    b. Angiography
    c. PET scan
    d. MRI

92. Select the purpose of a Veress needle insertion during a laparoscopic cholecystectomy:
    a. To anesthetize the patient's skin
    b. To inject CO_2 gas into the patient's abdominal cavity
    c. To irrigate the patient's abdomen
    d. To remove excess bile from the patient

93. Identify the maximum insufflation pressure during a laparoscopic cholecystectomy:
    a. 10 mm/Hg
    b. 21 mm/Hg
    c. 15 mm/Hg
    d. 12 mm/Hg

94. Identify the most common procedure performed by a general surgeon:
    a. Cholecystectomy
    b. Laparotomy
    c. Hysterectomy
    d. Herniorrhaphy

95. Choose the cleanser AORN recommends for showering a preoperative patient:
    a. Dove soap
    b. Povidone iodine
    c. Chlorhexidine gluconate (CHG)
    d. Alcohol

96. As you transport your Gynecology patient out of the O.R. after a procedure, the drainage bag from her indwelling catheter detaches from the cart and drops to the floor. Choose your best reaction:
    a. Reattach the drainage bag to a lower section of the cart
    b. Place the drainage bag on your patient's abdomen temporarily, until you get to the Post Anesthesia Care Unit
    c. Clamp her catheter, detach the drainage bag, and finish the transport
    d. Clamp the drainage bag tubing, place the bag on top of your patient, and transport her

97. The reverse Trendelenburg position is a variation of the:
    a. Supine position, in which the patient's head is lower than his feet
    b. Prone position, in which the patient's head is higher than his feet
    c. Supine position, in which the patient's head is higher than his feet
    d. Lateral position, in which the patient's head rests on a pillow, level with his feet

98. Your patient is eight months pregnant. Her surgery requires a supine position. Indicate how best to prevent hypotension from uterine pressure on her aorta and vena cava:
    a. Raise your patient's legs onto pillows to prevent venous pooling
    b. Place a padded wedge under her right side
    c. Place a small pillow under her waist
    d. Apply sequential compression stockings to her lower legs

99. Choose the appropriate safety technique when placing your patient into the prone position:
    a. Move quickly to minimize stress on your patient's joints
    b. Move slowly to allow him time to adjust to the change in position
    c. Enlist at least four people to turn an adult patient from supine to prone
    d. B and C

100. Choose the appropriate method for transferring your patient from a stretcher onto an operating table:
    a. Lock the stretcher's wheels prior to moving your patient; the O.R. table is always locked, so do not check it
    b. Enlist at least two people for transfer: one to stabilize the stretcher, and one on the opposite side of the operating table to receive your patient
    c. If your patient is awake, there is no need for a second person to receive him or her
    d. Raise the stretcher higher than the operating table, so your patient can move down onto the operating table independently

101. Choose the preferred method for shaving a male patient's abdomen prior to his surgical procedure:
    a. Shave him with a razor, warm water, and antiseptic soap
    b. Shave him with a razor on dry skin
    c. Use electric clippers to shave his abdomen
    d. Use hot wax to remove his hair

102. Choose the best location to shave your patient, so his hair removal occurs as close to the time of surgery as possible:
    a. In the O.R., as part of the prep
    b. In the Holding Area
    c. In your patient's hospital room
    d. In the hallway outside the O.R.

103. You are the circulating nurse on a major case. The scrub nurse requests more lap sponges. Since you are phoning Pathology, you quickly pass the sponges, but allow the scrub nurse to count them while you relay the report to the surgeon. Choose the TRUE statement regarding this action:
    a. Both the scrub nurse and the circulating nurse must witness the sponge count
    b. You should quickly count with the scrub nurse, and then relay the Pathology report to the surgeon
    c. The scrub nurse may count the sponges alone, providing she speaks loudly
    d. A and B

104. Choose the correct order for the scrub nurse's sponge count:
    a. First count the sponges on the Mayo stand, then the sponges on the surgical field
    b. First count the sponges nearest the patient's incision, secondly the sponges on sticks, thirdly sponges on the Mayo stand, and finally the sponges on the back table
    c. First count unopened packs on the back table, secondly sponges on the Mayo stand, and finally the surgical field, including sponge sticks
    d. First count the circulating nurse's soiled sponges, secondly the surgical field and sponge sticks, thirdly the Mayo stand, and finally the back table

105. Choose the correct reaction for the circulating nurse who finds the sponge count is incorrect following an open abdominal procedure:
    a. Inform the surgeon and anesthesiologist; call Radiology for an abdominal x-ray
    b. Inform the surgeon; send the patient to the Post Anesthesia Care Unit (PACU); and continue to search for the sponge
    c. Send the patient to the PACU; continue to search for the sponge; if it is not found, file an Incident Report
    d. Call your supervisor; send the patient to the PACU; continue to search; if the sponge is not found, inform patient's family

106. Choose the conditions that require you to change the dispersive electrode (Bovie pad) site:
    a. Scar tissue, excessive adipose tissue, or metal prosthetic implant
    b. Bony prominence, pacemaker, or automatic cardiac defibrillator
    c. Abundant muscle tissue or tanned skin
    d. A and B

107. While prepping your patient for electrosurgery, you notice the dispersive electrode pad is a different brand than the cautery machine. Choose your most appropriate action:
    a. Call Central Sterilizing or check the supply room for a matching dispersive pad
    b. Use the pad you have; they are all interchangeable
    c. Inform the surgeon and give him a hand-held cautery device that does not require a dispersive electrode
    d. Place the dispersive electrode pad on the patient, without attaching it to the generator

108. Choose the most appropriate needle for tissue that is difficult to penetrate:
    a. Taper-point
    b. Cutting-point
    c. Blunt-tip
    d. Saber-tip

109. Identify the most commonly used passive drain:
    a. Jackson Pratt
    b. Penrose
    c. Hemovac
    d. Sump

110. Identify the TRUE statement regarding a Jackson Pratt (JP) and a Hemovac drain:
    a. JP and Hemovac are the only closed systems that minimize bacteria entering the wound, and permit accurate drainage measurement
    b. They are simple-lumened drains that lie flat under the dressing
    c. They are double-lumened drains that can be attached to external suction
    d. A JP drains a surgical site of small amounts of fluid and blood, whereas the larger Hemovac is both a drain and a device for autologous retransfusion

111. Identify the method the anesthesiologist uses to verify proper placement of the patient's endotracheal tube:
    a. Observing fog in the laryngoscope
    b. Listening to the lungs for bilateral breath sounds
    c. Watching end-tidal oxygen (O2) levels
    d. Inspecting the oral cavity

112. Choose the correct method for assisting the anesthesiologist during intubation:
    a. Pull outwardly on the corner of the patient's mouth to enhance visualization of the vocal chords
    b. Inflate the balloon on the endotracheal tube with 1 mL of air
    c. Hold the endotracheal tube for easy access by the anesthesiologist
    d. A and C

113. Select the items the perioperative nurse has standing by for vomitus, in case the patient was not NPO prior to surgery:
    a. Nasogastric tube and emesis basin
    b. Suction catheter with a soft tip
    c. Sterile towels
    d. A and B

114. Identify the weak anesthesia gas that supplements other inhalation agents and narcotics:
    a. Isoflurane
    b. Desflurane
    c. Nitrous oxide
    d. Sevoflurane

115. The best method to prevent your patient's exhaled anesthetic gases from contaminating the O.R.'s atmosphere is a:
    a. CO2 system
    b. Scavenger system connected to a suction line
    c. Filtration system
    d. Reservoir bag

116. Identify the surgical team's signs and symptoms when there is exhaled anesthetic gas in the O.R.:
    a. Dizziness, nausea, and headaches
    b. Fatigue, drowsiness, and decreased mental acuity
    c. Hyperactivity, diaphoresis, and decreased body temperature
    d. A and B

117. Identify the iatrogenic diseases caused by exposure to anesthetic gases:
    a. Leukemia and heart disease
    b. Miscarriages and reduced fertility
    c. Liver, renal, and neurological diseases
    d. B and C

118. Select the equipment you must prepare for an orthopedic case with a Bier Block:
    a. Two tourniquets or one double-cuffed tourniquet, an Esmarch bandage, and a local anesthetic
    b. A spinal tray, extra pillows, a leg holder, an Esmarch bandage, and a local anesthetic
    c. An epidural catheter, a local anesthetic, and prep solution
    d. Xylocaine, a 20 mL syringe, prep solution, a blood pressure monitor, and a pulse oximeter

119. Identify the FALSE responsibility of the circulating nurse:
    a. Transporting the patient into the Operating Room
    b. Taking report from the Holding Area nurse
    c. Relaying patient information to other perioperative staff
    d. Passing instruments to the surgeon during surgery

120. Identify the TRUE responsibility of the circulating nurse to the patient's family when surgery is prolonged:
    a. Your only obligations are to the patient
    b. Call into the Waiting Room to inform the family about the patient's condition, and to relay updates from the surgeon
    c. Go to the Waiting Room in person to check on the family and to give them updates
    d. Go to the waiting room to offer the family coffee

121. Identify the Joint Commission's targeted solution for reducing patient injuries that result from poor communication between caregivers:
    a. A standardized hand-off procedure
    b. Preoperative instructions for patients to read
    c. Safety standards for Holding Area staff
    d. Marking the surgical site

122. Identify the scrub nurse's duty when receiving sponges, sharps or sutures with needles:
a. Tell the surgeon to wait for his next instrument and immediately count these items with the circulating nurse
b. Count these items with the circulating nurse as soon as possible after receiving them
c. Keep these items unopened on the back table, until there is time to open and count them
d. B and C

123. Identify the team members who co-sign the Perioperative Report to verify that the sponge, sharps and instrument counts were correct:
a. The surgeon and the circulating nurse
b. The scrub nurse and the circulating nurse
c. The anesthetist and circulating nurse
d. A and B

124. Select the information the nurse must document when a tourniquet is used during surgery:
a. An assessment of the skin above the tourniquet, and the type of skin protection used under the cuff
b. The tourniquet's location, cuff pressure, calibration, and times of inflation and deflation
c. The cuff material and the condition of the opposite limb for comparison
d. The calibration pressure and the equipment's usage history

125. Choose the information that the circulating nurse does NOT document:
a. Amount of prep solution
b. Type and amount of irrigation
c. Fluid output
d. Blood products

126. Choose the observations the perioperative nurse records when monitoring a patient who receives local anesthesia:
a. Skin color and condition; mental status; anesthetic dose; and temperature
b. Blood pressure; pulse rate and rhythm; respirations; and O2 saturation
c. Exact site of each local injection and time elapsed for anesthesia
d. A and B

127. Select the most probable nursing diagnosis for a patient receiving local anesthetic, who complains of dizziness, tremors, and visual disturbances:
a. Epilepsy
b. Toxic reaction to local anesthetic
c. Hypoglycemia from NPO order
d. Excessively bright overhead lights

128. Select your most appropriate response to your patient's adverse reaction to local anesthetic:
a. Inform the surgeon; establish and maintain an airway; and administer O2
b. Ask the anesthesiologist for assistance; administer a sedative; and bring the Crash Cart
c. Administer Narcan
d. A and B

129. Choose the information regarding the patient's position the nurse must document:
    a. Skin condition before and after surgery; type and placement of positioning equipment; team members who positioned the patient; and changes in position
    b. Height of the operating table and Mayo stand
    c. Number of perioperative staff assisting the surgeon
    d. A and B

130. Identify the standard information required to hand-off a surgical patient:
    a. The patient's position during surgery and the prep solution
    b. The patient name, age, sex, type of anesthesia, and estimated blood loss
    c. The type of surgical procedure, and the surgeon's and anesthetist's names
    d. B and C

131. Select the medication identification requirement for the scrub nurse:
    a. Use pre-printed medication labels
    b. Store drugs in different types of containers to simplify identification
    c. When pre-printed labels are unavailable, label drugs with a sterile marker
    d. A and C

132. Your patient's mole was sent to Pathology for a frozen section. Your patient becomes very anxious while awaiting the biopsy report. The surgeon verbally orders you to administer 10 mg of Valium orally. Choose the correct verification method:
    a. Write the order on a paper or white board; show it to the surgeon for confirmation
    b. Confirm it with the scrub nurse
    c. Check the patient's record for drug allergies
    d. Check the patient's record for drug orders

133. Identify the food or drink that a GI patient must avoid for the first three weeks post-operatively:
    a. Citrus fruits
    b. Green vegetables
    c. Carbonated beverages
    d. Dairy products

134. Identify the FALSE information for discharge instructions:
    a. Include the patient's medication instructions, dosage, schedule, diet, and physician's phone number
    b. Include the patient's wound care, signs of infection, and symptoms that require a call to a physician or a nurse practitioner
    c. Tell the patient when to make an appointment for follow-up care
    d. Remind the patient to call a physician or nurse practitioner if the wound itches or prickles

135. Your patient calls Ambulatory Surgery five days after a laparoscopic procedure with general anesthetic, complaining of a persistent cough. Choose your best response:
    a. Advise her to splint over the incision to eliminate pain when coughing
    b. Ask if she has a fever
    c. Advise her to call her physician's office
    d. Ask if her cough is productive, and tell her how to achieve postural drainage

136. Choose the best method to confirm your patient understands his discharge instructions:
    a. Have your patient complete a competency quiz
    b. Have your patient "teach back" the instructions to you
    c. Ask your patient if he has any questions
    d. Give your patient a postoperative instruction booklet

137. Identify the critical danger sign(s) for a liver, biliary tract, pancreas or spleen post-op patient to report to the physician:
    a. Fever of 38.3° C (101° F)
    b. Chills
    c. Increase abdominal swelling or pain
    d. Redness, swelling, and purulent drainage from the incision

138. Identify the surgical patients who are NOT high-risk for developing Methicillin-Resistant Staphylococcus Aureus (MRSA):
    a. High-risk patients with underlying diseases
    b. Patients with prolonged hospitalizations
    c. Patients from the Intensive Care Unit
    d. Patients from the Same Day Surgery unit

139. Identify the oldest, safest, least expensive, and best understood sterilization method:
    a. Ethylene oxide
    b. Steam
    c. Dry heat
    d. Hydrogen Peroxide Gas Plasma

140. Flash sterilization differs from terminal sterilization because:
    a. Flash sterilization is inappropriate for sterile storage
    b. A single wrapper may be appropriate for certain types of instruments, per the manufacturer's instructions
    c. Terminal sterilization requires at least 10 minutes of drying time
    d. A and B

141. The proper testing technique to determine if effective sterilization occurred is a:
    a. Biological indicator containing known, living, highly resistant spores
    b. Chemical indicator, which changes in color
    c. Thermal indicator, which changes in color
    d. Bacterial vial with live bacteria

142. Choose the trait that is NOT an advantage of steam sterilization:
    a. Readily available
    b. Leaves no toxic residue
    c. Compatible with all materials
    d. Fast

143. Choose the process that kills pathogenic microorganisms through the application of liquid chemical germicides:
   a. Sterilization
   b. Disinfection
   c. Purification
   d. Fumigation

144. Identify the infectious agent that causes Creutzfeldt-Jakob disease (CJD or mad cow disease):
   a. Bacteria
   b. Virus
   c. Enzyme
   d. Prion

145. The best place to find an up-to-date protocol for sterilizing instruments that contact a CJD patient's nerve or eye tissue is your:
   a. Facility's Policy & Procedure Manual
   b. Center for Disease Control and World Health Organization
   c. County Health Department
   d. State Health Department

146. The infectious bacteria usually transferred to a wound from hair is:
   a. Streptococcus
   b. Staphylococcus
   c. MRSA
   d. E-coli

147. Indicate the factor that increases the surgical patient's risk of infection:
   a. Obesity
   b. Previous joint replacement
   c. Radiation therapy
   d. A and C

148. Choose your best response to a new perioperative nurse wearing pink nail polish while scrubbing:
   a. Explain to her that she must remove her nail polish prior to scrubbing
   b. Do nothing; the nail polish does not pose a problem
   c. Report her to the supervisor for wearing nail polish
   d. Replace her with someone who has no nail polish

149. Choose your best response when you drop a sterile, single-use item on the floor and do not have a replacement for it:
   a. Flash sterilize it
   b. Send it to CSS for reprocessing
   c. Soak it in alkaline glutaraldehyde for 20 minutes
   d. Cancel the case

150. Choose your best response when a pointed towel clip securing a drape unfastens:
    a. Remove the towel clip and replace it with another one
    b. If the towel clip is visible, re-clasp it
    c. Ignore the towel clip
    d. Ask the circulating nurse to remove the towel clip

151. Identify the areas of a sterile gown that are contaminated after donning:
    a. Cuffs, sleeves above the elbow, and panels below the waist
    b. Panels below the waist, back, and lower arms
    c. Neckline, shoulder, cuffs, and axillae (underarms)
    d. Cuffs to 2" above the elbow, cuffs, neckline, and axillae (underarms)

152. Identify the correct technique for opening a sterile item:
    a. First, open the flap closest to you
    b. Once opened, allow all flaps to hang freely
    c. First, open the flap farthest away from you
    d. Open heavy items first, then toss them onto stacked towels

153. You are circulating nurse on a case that requires a large amount of irrigation solution. You dispense 1,000 mL of sterile NSS, and then add 500 mL more as the case progresses. Since you only have 1,000 mL screw-top containers, choose the correct way to handle the 500 mL excess saline:
    a. Replace the cap and save it for adding later
    b. Leave the cap off and save it for adding later
    c. Save it by handing the scrub nurse an additional bowl and pouring the remainder in it
    d. Discard it; once poured, the saline is contaminated

154. Identify the appropriate safety precaution for unscrubbed personnel working in a sterile setup.
    a. Never walk between sterile fields
    b. Keep a safe distance from sterile fields
    c. Keep your back to sterile fields
    d. A and B

155. Identify the ventilation system that provides unidirectional, filtered, bacteria-free air circulation:
    a. Uni-air Flow System
    b. Laminair Air Flow System
    c. Hepa-flow System
    d. Ortho-flow System

156. Identify the safety feature necessary for materials used in the Operating Room:
    a. Smooth and nonporous surface
    b. Easily cleaned, washable surface
    c. Ridged surface to prevent falls
    d. A and B

157. Choose the most likely effect on the O.R. of a high school class observing a case, with the patient's permission:
    a. Improved public relations and increased interest in surgical careers
    b. Increased microorganism colonies from increased traffic
    c. Increased risk of surgical site infection (SSI)
    d. B and C

158. Identify the O.R. surfaces that require the most attention from cleaners:
    a. Vertical surfaces
    b. Horizontal surfaces
    c. Metal surfaces
    d. Glass surfaces

159. Select the most appropriate disinfectant to use in the O.R. prior to the first surgery of the day:
    a. Alcohol
    b. Formalin
    c. Hospital-grade disinfectant approved by the EPA
    d. Immerse in 1N Sodium hydroxide (NaOH) in a covered pan for one hour, steam autoclave for 30 minutes at 121°C, AND subject to routine sterilization

160. Select the best time to schedule surgery for a patient who is infected with a known airborne-transmitted disease:
    a. First case in the morning
    b. Any time
    c. Last case of the day
    d. Do not schedule, until this patient is disease-free

161. Identify the special care requirements for ophthalmic instruments:
    a. Gently hand wash them
    b. Closely examine their tips before use
    c. Send them to CSS for processing
    d. A and B

162. Choose the best method for transferring contaminated instruments to Central Sterile Supply (CSS):
    a. Transport contaminated instruments sealed in a closed container, cart, or plastic bag
    b. Transport contaminated instruments on an open cart
    c. Transport contaminated instruments in a large basin, submerged in water
    d. Transport contaminated instruments covered in a used drape

163. You opened a set of special instruments onto a ring stand before surgery began, but they were untouched during this case. Choose your appropriate action regarding these instruments following surgery:
    a. Cover them for use in the next case; they were not touched and remain sterile
    b. Once opened during surgery, instruments require reprocessing by CSS
    c. Instruct the scrub nurse to re-wrap them and seal them with tape
    d. A and C

164. Identify the gloving technique that poses the greatest risk of contamination to the scrub nurse:
    a. Closed technique
    b. Open technique
    c. Gloved by other scrub personnel
    d. Double gloving

165. Choose the appropriate action for a member of the scrub team whose glove is contaminated:
    a. Step away from the sterile field, have the circulating nurse remove the contaminated glove, and don sterile gloves
    b. Step away from the sterile field, have the circulating nurse remove the contaminated glove and gown, then don a sterile gown and gloves
    c. Leave the sterile area, scrub, then don a sterile gown and gloves
    d. Step away from sterile field, and don a sterile glove over the contaminated glove

166. Choose the appropriate technique for the circulating nurse to remove a contaminated glove from a member of the surgical team:
    a. Pull the gown cuff down over your co-worker's hand
    b. Do not pull down the gown cuff
    c. Grasp the contaminated glove close to your co-worker's wrist, remove it inside out, and discard it
    d. A and C

167. Select the safety precaution the circulating nurse uses before removing a contaminated glove from a member of the surgical team:
    a. Don sterile gloves
    b. Don clean gloves
    c. Use care not to contaminate your co-worker's gown or remaining glove
    d. B and C

168. Identify the safety precaution the scrub nurse takes when preparing for invasive surgery:
    a. Double-glove
    b. Wear an x-ray apron under the sterile gown
    c. Wear high booties over shoes
    d. Wear a laser high-filtration mask

169. Identify the most common complication the patient may sustain during extubation:
    a. Vomiting (emesis)
    b. Laryngospasm and/or bronchospasm
    c. Hyperventilation
    d. A and B

170. Most O.R. fires that injure the patient occur in the:
    a. Abdominal area, from electrosurgery sparks
    b. Facial area, due to its high oxygen concentration
    c. Intra-abdominal area during laparoscopic laser usage
    d. Perineal area, from electrosurgery or laser usage

171. Select the best fire extinguisher for O.R. use:
    a. Carbon dioxide
    b. Halon
    c. Pressurized water
    d. Sodium bicarbonate

172. Identify the heat-generating equipment that must not contact the patient's drape, in case its connectors detach:
    a. Fiber-optic cords
    b. Electrosurgery cords
    c. Suction tubing
    d. Laser cords

173. Select the nurse's first and foremost action when a fire engulfs the surgical patient's drapes:
    a. Get the fire extinguisher
    b. Sound the fire alarm
    c. Remove the drapes from the patient
    d. Announce "Code Red"

174. To activate the fire extinguisher, the nurse must:
    a. Pull the pin
    b. Squeeze the handle
    c. Aim the spray at the top of the fire, and sweep it downward
    d. A and B

175. Identify the safety measure used in the O.R. to prevent fires:
    a. Never use less than 100% oxygen during facial surgery
    b. Shave all beards and mustaches prior to facial surgery
    c. Remove unnecessary foot pedals from around surgeon's feet
    d. Keep the electrosurgery pencil on the field, so the surgeon can reach it easily
176. Select the correct safety precaution for laser use:
    a. Place the laser on 'ready' when it is not in use
    b. Position wet towels around the patient's incision site
    c. Use non-reflective instruments to avoid arcing
    d. B and C

177. Identify the drug of choice for malignant hyperthermia patients:
    a. Dantrolene sodium (Dantrium)
    b. Succinylcholine (Anectine)
    c. Fentanyl
    d. Morphine

178. Select the items the nurse collects to treat malignant hyperthermia:
a. Thirty-six or more vials of Dantrolene sodium (Dantrium); enough preservative-free sterile injectable water to reconstitute the Dantrium; sodium bicarbonate; and a new anesthesia machine, if possible
b. A protocol sheet for reference; cold sterile NSS for wound irrigation; cold IV solution; ice or a cooling blanket for surface cooling; cold gastric and rectal lavage equipment; a new anesthesia circuit and carbon dioxide absorbent; and Vacutainer blood tubes for specimen testing
c. A warming blanket; sequential stockings; warm NSS; warm IV solutions; a new anesthesia machine or circuits and carbon dioxide absorbent
d. A and B

179. Choose your best response when a preoperative patient tells you he developed a high fever during his last surgical procedure:
a. Explain to your patient that his elevated temperature was more than likely due to an infection, and that if it recurs during this procedure, the anesthesiologist will administer antibiotics
b. Page the anesthesiologist and the surgeon; ask them if they want to order a muscle biopsy and precautions for malignant hyperthermia
c. Comfort the patient by telling him the O.R. is cooled by air conditioning set on "low", and the anesthesiologist will monitor his body temperature at all times
d. Explain that his body temperature may have risen as a response to the cool O.R., and then give the patient a warm blanket

180. Identify the resource you must read following a large Formalin spill on your surgical scrubs, to find out its hazards and appropriate first aid:
a. OSHA
b. SDS
c. NIOSH
d. FDA

181. Select the appropriate safety precautions when working with methyl methacrylate:
a. Do not wear contact lenses
b. Do not use electronic equipment while mixing
c. Pour the powder into the liquid
d. A and B

182. Identify the competency that is NOT a minimum qualification for an O.R. supervisor:
a. Managerial skills
b. Clinical expertise
c. Central Sterilization techniques expertise
d. Interpersonal skills

183. Identify the cost-saving technique below:
a. Efficient turn-over of the Operating Room between cases
b. Staff skipping breaks, except for lunch
c. Reusing laser glasses, even if they are scratched
d. Recapping sterile NSS irrigation for reuse in other cases

184. Choose the important consideration for scheduling cases in the O.R.:
    a. Staffing availability
    b. Specialty room availability (e.g., for an open heart case)
    c. Lunch schedule
    d. A and B

185. Select the first step for the committee to choose new sterile drapes for the O.R.:
    a. Compare drape costs from one manufacturer to another
    b. Establish requirements for the new drapes
    c. Call at least three manufacturer's sales representatives to set up demonstrations
    d. Check the material for fire resistance and thickness

186. Identify the decisions that are included in the nurse's Five Rights of Delegation:
    a. Right task, right circumstances, and right person
    b. Right communication and right supervision
    c. Right diagnosis and right status
    d. A and B

187. Identify the emphasis of the Perioperative Patient Focused Model:
    a. The outcome-driven nature of perioperative patient care
    b. Implementation of the care plan
    c. Prevention of injury
    d. Elimination of risk

188. Choose the practice that fits this definition: "The systematic, meticulous process used to identify an issue, to gather and assess the best evidence, to draft and employ a practice change, and to evaluate the process."
    a. Evidence-based practice
    b. Advanced nursing practice
    c. Quality-assurance practice
    d. Risk-reduction practice

189. Performance improvement efforts attempt to:
    a. Improve quality
    b. Improve effectiveness
    c. Increase the number of surgeries
    d. A and B

190. Identify the responsibilities of the surgical team members who wear sterile attire:
    a. Take directions from the surgeon
    b. Set up non-sterile equipment
    c. Assist the anesthetist during induction
    d. Position the anesthetized patient

191. Select the tasks delegated to the perioperative nurse in the role of the circulator:
    a. Coordinating care of the surgical patient
    b. Patient advocacy during the intraoperative period
    c. Managing and implementing activities on the sterile field
    d. A and B

192. The circulating nurse stands by the patient during induction to assist the anesthetist and:
    a. Offer emotional support to the patient
    b. Prevent patient falls
    c. Observe the sterile set-up
    d. A and B

193. Choose the factors the nurse manager considers when making scrub assignments for the following day's surgeries:
    a. Necessary expertise
    b. Staffing skill mix
    c. Seniority
    d. A and B

194. Identify the purpose of physician preference cards:
    a. Lists the physician's preferred sutures, dressings, special instruments, and equipment
    b. Lists the surgeon's phone number for questions
    c. Lists every instrument the surgeon may need
    d. Lists the physician's preferred staff

195. Choose the information that the circulating nurse is NOT responsible for recording:
    a. Temperature of the Operating Room
    b. Incision time
    c. End of surgery time
    d. Anesthesia induction time

196. Choose the method the perioperative nurse uses to alleviate patient anxiety and fear preoperatively:
    a. Attentive listening
    b. Reassurance
    c. Telling the patient that there is nothing to fear
    d. A and B

197. Select the equipment required by the nurse to monitor a patient receiving local anesthetic:
    a. Blood pressure monitor and resuscitation equipment
    b. Electrocardiograph and oximeter
    c. Anesthesia machine
    d. A and B

198. Identify the perioperative personnel who must sign sponge counts:
    a. Circulating nurse
    b. Scrub nurse
    c. Surgeon
    d. A and B

199. Identify the danger posed when the nurse positions the overhead lights for the upcoming surgery, prior to bringing the patient into the Operating Room:
    a. Head injuries
    b. Time-savings
    c. Contamination
    d. Added anxiety for the patient

200. Identify the major reason contributing to nurses leaving their profession:
    a. Infectious disease exposure
    b. Early work hours
    c. Workplace occupational hazards
    d. Difficult surgeons

Answer Key and Explanations

1. D: Essential perioperative patient assessment includes: Allergies, especially to medications or latex; implants or pacemakers, which affect coagulation during electrocautery; and confirmation of the type and location of the proposed surgery. Age and weight are important for anesthesia, but an approximation is sufficient. *Exact* age and weight are unnecessary.

2. A: Ace bandages and IV tubing contain latex to make them stretchy. Symptoms of latex allergies are redness, rash, and asthmatic reactions on contact. Notify the surgeon and anesthetist immediately. Bronchitis is unlikely because the patient's History and Physical showed no respiratory disease. Since wheezing began *after* IV insertion, its most likely cause is an allergic reaction. Normal saline solution rarely causes any type of negative reaction. Fear of surgery is common, but usually presents as anxiety.

3. B: Standard procedure is for the nurse to ask the patient, parent, or guardian to clearly point out the surgery site, and ensure the surgeon marked the same position with a permanent marker. Sticky notes and adhesive tape dislodge easily when wet with sweat, blood, and irrigation fluids. One legal requirement of the preoperative assessment is confirming that the surgical permit agrees with the patient's description of the location and type of surgical procedure. If the permit differs from the patient's description of the proposed procedure, the nurse contacts the surgeon, and confirms the proper procedure and site with *both* the surgeon and patient, parent, or guardian.

4. C: Only the surgeon who performs the procedure marks the site.

5. D: The perioperative nurse performs a variety of functions, including patient assessment and development of a nursing diagnosis. During the perioperative phase, the nurse assembles pertinent patient information, identifies desired outcomes, then develops and executes a plan of care.

6. C: The nurse ignores the patient's insurance and financial status because they could prejudice his care. Leave billing to the Admissions clerk. Concentrate instead on the three major components of the nursing assessment: (1) your patient's diagnosis, current physical condition (including allergies), and psychosocial status; (2) his history of hospital stays, major illnesses, and previous surgeries; and (3) the scheduled surgical procedure, your patient's understanding of it, and your proposed plan of care.

7. D: The type of glove used by the surgical technologist determines her latex exposure level. If she noticed a latex reaction, such as rash after removal of the gloves, it could indicate a potentially lethal latex allergy. Her area of specialization is unimportant for her safety, so asking her about it would just serve as an icebreaker.

8. A: The preoperative patient facing a breast biopsy experiences the fear of body image change (disfigurement), in addition to more common fears associated with surgery and anesthesia. Apprehension associated with surgical intervention and anesthesia include, but are not limited to, possible surgical outcomes, lifestyle effects, loss of control, pain, and death.

9. D: When you discover that your perioperative patient is anxious, allay her apprehension with the proper nursing intervention: Listen attentively, provide reassurance, encourage her to express her

anxiety or fear, then address it, and provide emotional support. Explaining every surgical detail would only increase her level of apprehension.

10. B: TPR, skin appearance, and level of consciousness are parts of the physical assessment, not the psychosocial assessment. Psychosocial assessment means estimating your patient's: Capacity to understand the surgical procedure; coping ability; comprehension and inclination to learn; anxiety level regarding the procedure and outcome; knowledge of perioperative practices; and cultural or spiritual beliefs, as they relate to the procedure.

11. A: Determine the cause of your patient's knowledge deficit before surgery. Consider a language barrier, impaired communication skills, low mental capacity, or a lack of information regarding the surgical procedure. Your patient's education level does not influence his intelligence level.

12. D: Risk factors for deep vein thrombosis (DVT) include age older than 50, a history of varicose veins, myocardial infarction, atrial fibrillation, cancer, ischemic stroke, previous DVT, diabetes, obesity, paralysis, and inhibitor deficiency state. A history of ovarian cysts does not increase the risk of DVT.

13. C: Graduated compression stockings (sequential stockings) prevent deep vein thrombosis. Correct positioning inhibits the formation of pressure sores. Good sterile technique helps prevent infections. Proper grounding techniques and education on the correct usage of O.R. equipment help avoid electrical injury.

14. B: Identify the patient, take report from the Holding Area nurse, review the Assessment sheet and any test results, then transport the patient.

15. D: The perioperative nurse must understand anatomy, surgical procedures, instruments and O.R. equipment. The anesthesiologist or nurse anesthetist performs endotracheal tube insertion. The perioperative nurse assists with intubation, but is not responsible for identifying internal physical landmarks to ensure tube placement is correct.

16. B: A "never event" is an adverse occurrence that is plainly identifiable and measurable, results in death or major disability, and is generally preventable. "Never events" include: Surgery performed on the wrong body part or wrong patient; incorrect procedure; retention of a foreign object following surgery; medication error or contaminated drug; inappropriate equipment use; IV air embolism; incompatible blood transfusion; stage 3 or 4 decubitus ulcers from improper positioning; wrong inhalation agent; a burn, fall, or death of an American Society of Anesthesiologists Class 1 patient.

17. C: Anxiety produces *slight* hypertension, increased pulse and respiratory rates, and is normal before any stressful event, such as surgery. Hypertension, COPD, and heart disease should appear in the Medical History section of the patient's *Preassessment Information Sheet.*

18. D: Ask your patient if he has any questions regarding the surgical procedure. Explain the procedure and post-operative expectations suitably for your patient's level of comprehension; avoid medical jargon. A practiced set of answers for each surgical procedure may help you feel prepared, but may sound too rehearsed to your patient. Each patient is unique. Customize your answers to your patient's specific learning abilities.

19. A: Emergency surgery, unusual time pressures, multiple patients entering O.R. suites simultaneously, and several procedures performed on each patient, are all factors that may contribute to selecting the wrong patient, body part, side, level, site or procedure.

20. A: Sometimes an anxious, premedicated patient answers to a wrong name, or two patients have the same or similar names. The *best* method to confirm your patient's identity is to check the wristband, confirm that it matches the name and unique number on the chart, and ask the patient (or parent/guardian) to spell the name. The Holding Area nurse may assist you with patient identification, but you must still check the chart, the wristband, and ask the patient to say his name.

21. D: Use the "time out" prior to starting the surgical procedure to verify your patient's identify, ensure the correct procedure is on record and verbally understood, the right site is marked, and all surgical implants are readily available (if applicable). Surgical staff only take breaks when relieved by other qualified staff members.

22. D: The grass allergy is irrelevant to the surgical procedure, unless it is performed in the field. Paralysis is important for positioning and for transferring the patient. The history and location of implants are relevant when using electrocoagulation.

23. D: Use the mnemonic device "I pass (the) baton" to recall the important steps for receiving a patient from the Holding Area:
(I) Introduction, explanation of your role
(P) Patient identification
(A) Assessment
(S) Situation (status)
(S) Safety concerns
(B) Background
(A) Actions taken or required
(T) Timing
(O) Ownership (responsible parties)
(N) Next (plan what happens next)

24. A: The Universal Protocol for prevention of wrong site, wrong procedure or wrong person surgeries has three steps:

(1) *Preoperative verification process,* which assures that all relevant test results and documents are available before the procedure begins, have been reviewed, and are consistent with the planned procedure.
(2) *Marking of the operative site* with a permanent marker, after verifying the location and procedure with the patient, family member or other responsible party is extremely important. This mark must remain visible after the patient's prep and draping for surgery.
(3) Taking a "time out" in the O.R. immediately prior to starting the surgical procedure, to verify the correct identity of the patient, the exact site of the proposed incision, the right scheduled procedure, and the availability of implants, if applicable.

25. A: Any penetrable, sterile package is contaminated if it shows any evidence of dampness. *When in doubt, throw it out!* Unwrap the tray, so it will not be used. Send the entire contents back to Central Sterile Supply for re-sterilization (reprocessing). Once the tray is wet, bacteria enter it. Allowing it to air dry does not re-sterilize it. Opening the tray on a ring stand does not change the fact that the tray and its contents are contaminated.

26. D: Freedom from infection is an extremely important desired outcome. Excellent aseptic technique, including the proper prepping of the incision site, contributes to the desired outcome of freedom from infection. The anesthetic agent itself does not have a major effect on the incidence of infection.

27. B: Sterile packages require pressure-sensitive chemical indicator tape that is specific to the type of sterilization technique (steam, dry heat, or gas). Black stripes appear on the autoclave tape when the pack is correctly sterilized. Surgical adhesive, paper tape, and water resistant tape are inappropriate for use on a sterile package.

28. A: Wrapping materials used during the sterilization process must meet certain safety standards, such as resistance to tears, punctures and abrasions. Other requirements include: Enough porosity to allow for steam or gas penetration and venting; effective air and microorganism barrier; secure enclosure of contents; moisture resistance (*not water-proof*); absence of toxic ingredients and non-fast dyes; sufficient seal integrity; aseptic delivery of contents to the sterile field; correct labeling; adequate size for even content distribution; and ability to sustain the sterility of contents until opening.

29. D: Rigid containers weigh up to 10 pounds. Condensation may occur on the surfaces of a rigid container, contaminating the entire package (referred to as "wet pack"). Despite its two drawbacks, rigid packaging is durable and provides excellent defense against damage to the contents.

30. D: *Exogenous* sources of infection come from outside the body, including the environment and hospital personnel. The patient's skin flora provides an *endogenous* source of infection because it is always present.

31. C: AORN, CDC and the WHO all recommend *against* the use of artificial nails because they increase fungal and bacterial colonization of the hands. Perioperative personnel with artificial nails still harbor Gram-negative microorganisms and yeasts, even after performing a preoperative surgical scrub correctly.

32. B: Normal flora are either symbiotic or commensal microorganisms that live on the patient's skin, mucous membranes, and hollow viscera. Poor aseptic technique, unclean equipment (including the overhead lights), and staff coughing, talking and breathing may lead to infection. However, the majority of surgical site infections are traced to the patient's own normal flora becoming pathogenic.

33. A: The three modes of transmission for microorganisms include droplet, airborne and contact. Body fluids, purulent material, blood, sneezing, coughing, talking, and dirty equipment are possible sources of contamination, which are included under the three modes of transmission.

34. D: Assume all patients are infectious and wear the correct Personal Protective Equipment (PPE). Universal Precautions were adopted by the Center for Disease Control (CDC) in 1987 to prevent the transmission of blood-borne pathogens, including but not limited to HIV and HBV. Universal Precautions pertain to blood and *any* body fluid that contains blood, such as semen, saliva, or vaginal secretions.

35. D: Universal precautions include proper hand washing techniques, careful handling of sharps (carefully passing pointed, hooked, or bladed instruments, and never recapping needles), and proper use of Personal Protective Equipment, such as gloves, masks, and gowns.

36. D: It is impossible to clear the skin entirely of microorganisms and spores. Even a strong antiseptic solution, such as povidone iodine, cannot make skin completely sterile, but just reduces the number of microorganisms. The purpose of aseptic practice is to prevent the invasion of microorganisms into the open incision, and to create and maintain the integrity of a sterile field surrounding the wound, isolating it from the merely clean adjacent areas.

37. B: The bronchoscopy procedure causes the patient to cough uncontrollably. Washings and brushings mean tiny tissue particles will become airborne. The risk of communicable disease means the O.R. staff must wear masks with shields, or masks with goggles.

38. B: *Never* shave the eyebrow. Use prep solution and carefully avoid getting it into the patient's eye. Apply ophthalmic ointment only if ordered to do so by the physician.

39. D: The length of time for a prep are determined by the manufacturer's recommendations and by expert studies of the effectiveness of the antimicrobial agents.

40. B: Once the drape slides off the surgical area, it becomes contaminated. The student nurse must remove the contaminated drape, discard it, and obtain a sterile replacement. Placing the contaminated drape on the sterile back table would contaminate the back table. Reprepping the surgical site is unnecessary; the draping material was originally sterile and only became contaminated when it shifted to the unprepped area.

41. C: The used surgical mask contains microorganisms from the nurse's respiratory tract and possibly from the patient. Remove the mask after surgery by handling its ties only, and then discard it into a covered container. *Never* hang a used mask around your neck, or place it in your pocket to reuse. When the mask hangs around the neck, the bacteria lose moisture and become an airborne source of contamination. Cost-savings are important, but we must not endanger the patient, visitors, or hospital personnel.

42. D: Ethylene oxide gas is toxic, flammable and explosive. It is carcinogenic and associated with reproductive problems. Therefore, its use is restricted to surgical items that cannot tolerate moist heat, such as rigid and flexible endoscopes, plastic items, fragile sharp instruments that would deteriorate with steam sterilization, and instruments with electrical components that would sustain damage when exposed to high moist heat.

43. A: When a unique instrument is contaminated during surgery, the circulating nurse dons gloves, retrieves the instrument, sanitizes it, flash sterilizes it, and returns it to the scrub nurse as quickly as possible. The circulating nurse wears gloves for protection against any blood-borne pathogens that may be on the instrument. Sanitizing the instrument removes visible debris only. A sterile towel is unnecessary for picking up a contaminated instrument. Flash sterilization is faster than sending the instrument to CSS. Alcohol and formaldehyde soaks are unacceptable sterilizing techniques.

44. D: Lift your patient's legs carefully, *slowly and in unison* to prevent injury to the sacroiliac joint.

45. B: Surgical preps begin at the incision site and moves outward in a spiral motion to the periphery. Most prep solutions require a 20-minute wait to ensure optimal killing of surface microorganisms.

46. B: Position the table strap 2 inches *above* the knees as soon as the patient moves onto the operating table. Remove the strap when the patient is ready for transport to the Recovery Room, and perioperative personnel are standing beside the patient for transfer assistance.

47. D: When returning your patient to the supine position from the lithotomy position, remove her feet from the stirrups, extend her legs completely to avoid abduction of the hips, close them, and then slowly lower them. Severe hypotension can result from lowering the legs too quickly, since 500 mL to 800 mL of blood diverts from the viscera to the lower extremities.

48. D: Jackknife position is used for many proctocological procedures. Jackknife is one of the most precarious positions. Your patient's mean arterial blood pressure may drop, due to venous pooling in the lower extremities and chest. A decrease in cardiac output and respirations may result from the restricted diaphragm movement.

49. A: Avoid metal implants in the circuit path between the active electrode and the dispersive electrode pad.

50. B: Use the needle holder to attach and remove blades to prevent injuries. Never touch the blade, or use the packaging to apply the blade to the handle. Toothed forceps would not create a firm grip on the blade.

51. B: Increasing power on the ultrasonic scalpel increases the cutting speed but decreases its coagulation capability. An ultrasonic scalpel vibrates at 55,000 times per second, allowing it to cut and coagulate simultaneously at temperatures lower than electrosurgery. The denatured protein creates a sticky coagulant.

52. C: The Army-Navy retractor is double-ended. A Weitlaner is a Balfour (self-retaining retractor) with a blade. The Army-Navy retractor does not contain a suction port.

53. A: Mersilene is a polyester fiber that is not absorbable. Chromic gut, Vicryl and plain surgical gut are absorbable sutures.

54. C: Surgical gut refers to suture that is derived from collagen found in the submucosal layer of the intestines of sheep, cattle or hogs. "Catgut" is a misnomer and may come from the Arabic word "kit", which means "dancing master's fiddle". Nylon suture is nonabsorbable.

55. D: Silk is prepared from thread spun by silkworm larvae. It is twisted or braided to increase its strength. It may be absorbed after several years.

56. D: Blunt suture-tip needles provide safer alternatives for prevention of percutaneous injuries in the OR. They are appropriate for use on internal tissue, not for use on skin closure. Blunt suture-tip needles come in a range of bluntness.

57. B: Pressing the staple firmly against the incision can cause unnecessary trauma. A better technique is to "kiss" the skin gently with the stapler when applying skin staples. Place staples ¼ inch apart.

58. D: *Shearing injuries* result when the tissue below the skin moves but the skin remains stationary. Shearing may be the consequence of pulling a patient instead of lifting him. The patient's subcutaneous capillaries tear, causing tissue ischemia, which may progress to a pressure ulcer. An inadequately padded bony prominence may also lead to a pressure ulcer after more than 20 minutes of direct weight-bearing, but this is an example of a *pressure injury*.

59. D: Any time the operating table position changes, the scrub nurse should adjust the Mayo stand to an appropriate height, taking care not to injure the patient. Never allow the Mayo stand to contact the patient. If a step stool improves your view of the surgical field better, request one.

60. A: Turn your immobile patient at least once every two hours to prevent pressure ulcers. Bony, weight-bearing areas like the heels, knees, hips, elbows, and buttocks are usually affected. High-risk patients include those with limited mobility, impaired cognition, diabetes, vascular disease, and vascular surgery.

61. D: Never use 100% oxygen (O_2) when assisting a facial surgeon because it increases the chances of a fire. Use a draping technique that does not allow pockets of O_2 to form. Oxygen that is trapped under the drape concentrates and becomes a fire hazard. Coat the patient's facial hair with a water-soluble lubricant during facial surgery, if the surgeon will employ any type of cautery.

62. D: Thrombin customarily comes from dried beef blood. Thrombin combines with fibrinogen to accelerate the coagulation process, and is useful for controlling capillary bleeding. Thrombin is dispensed as a white powder, which the scrub nurse mixes with sterile water or saline, and uses in conjunction with a gelatin sponge. Thrombin retains its potency for about three hours, but works best if used shortly after mixing. Thrombin is for *topical use only, never for injection*. Bovine-derived thrombin can lead to an autoimmune response, resulting in a severe bleeding complication.

63. C: Carbon dioxide (CO_2) lasers *can* damage the *cornea*. Water in the surface cells of the cornea absorbs the CO_2 laser's beam, resulting in an immediate, painful burn. Argon and Nd:YAG lasers can damage the *retina*. The lens of the eye refocuses the beam of the Argon and Nd: YAG laser and can damage the retina with no accompanying pain. Eye protection is very important during *any* procedure in which laser therapy is used, regardless of the gas. Even low levels of laser radiation can lead to permanent eye injury.

64. D: *Appropriate* eye-wear is necessary for all laser surgeries, even endoscopic. Laser glasses are specific to the type of laser used. Laser precautions include: Place "Danger, Laser Radiation" signs on all entrances to the O.R.; cover all windows; hang extra laser eye-wear outside the doors, so anyone entering will be protected; place wet gauze pads on the anesthetized patient's eyes; provide protective eye-wear for the conscious patient; and use nonreflective instruments.

65. B: The *McBurney incision* is an oblique, muscle-splitting incision that surgeons use for an open appendectomy.

66. C: A suprapubic incision is also called a Pfannenstiel. It is a gently curved, transverse incision, extending across the patient's lower abdomen, approximately 1cm above the *symphysis pubis*. Suprapubic incisions are commonly used for obstetric and gynecological procedures, such as elective Caesarean sections. The midabdominal transverse incision runs from slightly above the patient's umbilicus and extends laterally to the lumbar region. The subcostal is an oblique incision

that begins in the epigastrium and extends laterally at an oblique angle, ending slightly below the patient's costal margin.

67. A: A total gastrectomy results in an esophagojejunostomy.

68. A: Laparoscopy requires specialized surgical training and can usually only be used for elective surgery, not emergencies. However, it offers the patient many advantages, including: Decreased blood loss; reduced infection risk; increased return of GI function; diminished chance of small bowel obstruction; lowered risk of incisional hernia; and reduced postoperative pain.

69. D: Kitners, lap pads, RAY-TEC® sponges, peanuts, tonsil sponges and cottonoid patties are all countable items. Thrombin-soaked gelatin sponges are not countable, since the body absorbs them, and they control bleeding.

70. B: Formaldehyde is a proven carcinogen and a respiratory irritant that also causes watering of the eyes. Formaldehyde can fix contact lenses to the wearer's eyes. Perioperative nurses should wear gloves and use formaldehyde only under a fume hood, or at least in a well-ventilated area.

71. D: When electrosurgery or laser use results in surgical smoke, evacuate the smoke (plume) with suction that has an in-line filter. If a large amount of smoke is present, a free-standing smoke evacuator is required. Use laser (high particle filtration) to prevent air-borne contaminants from entering the respiratory systems of the perioperative staff. Never leave the O.R. doors open during any surgical procedure.

72. B: A clean wound (Class I) means the patient's GI, respiratory, or GU tract are intact (not entered). A clean contaminated wound (Class II) means the surgeon entered the patient's GI, respiratory, or GU tract by controlled means. A contaminated wound (Class III) is grossly (visibly) contaminated with a foreign substance, but there is no sign of infection. A dirty or infected wound (Class IV) means the surgical site contains infected or dead (necrotic) tissue.

73. B: When your bare thumb touched the sterile glove, the glove became contaminated. Scrubbing before donning a sterile gown and gloves removes some surface bacteria, but the skin is *never* completely sterile. Discard your contaminated gloves. Ask the circulating nurse to provide you with a new pair. Your hand is not contaminated, since what you touched was a sterile glove, but your skin contaminated your glove. There is no need to start over entirely, since only your glove is contaminated. Sterile saline cannot remove bacterial contamination from a glove.

74. C: Once you touch the faucet with your hand, you are contaminated. The appropriate action is to start your scrub over from the beginning, using a new scrub sponge or brush. Proceeding into the O.R. with a contaminated hand, rinsing for an extra minute, or double-gloving are unacceptable, high-risk actions. Your only safe choice is to begin again.

75. C: When you encounter another person who is "scrubbed in", you pass back-to-back. Your back is not considered sterile, so you should not turn your back to the O.R. table. Back-to-back is the best technique for passing.

76. B: Once a sterile field is set up, the perioperative staff must *continually* monitor it. A two-hour window between the opening of the sterile items and the start of surgery is acceptable. It would not be cost-effective to discard the sterile items and order new ones. The staff may leave the room *only* if someone who relieves them can continually monitor the sterile fields.

77. A: The Richardson, Army-Navy and Deaver are all retractors. The Allis, Babcock and Kocher are grasping clamps. The towel clip and sponge forceps are also grasping clamps. Metzenbaum, Mayo and Catroviejo are types of scissors.

78. B: The color code is yellow for air, green for oxygen, and blue for nitrous oxide. Gas fittings are not interchangeable, to prevent injuries.

79. A: "Memory" refers to any material, including sutures that tends to return to its original positioning or folding position. Gently stretch the memory suture, taking care not to create tension on its swaged needle.

80. B: Raise the patient's arm to allow for venous drainage, thereby preventing edema and necrosis later.

81. C: Remove the sterile 3" x3" gauze pads from the back table to eliminate their possible use in the current surgery. *Never* use a sponge on a sponge stick that does not have a radiopaque strip, in case it is retained and the patient must be reopened.

82. B: The circulating nurse should wear gloves or use a sponge stick to handle any sponge that comes from the surgical field. Microscopic contaminants are invisible, so even if the sponge appears clean, treat it as soiled. Your hospital policy determines if 5 or 10 sponges can accumulate, but the amount must be consistent. The circulator counts the sponges *with the scrub nurse,* then places them into a plastic bag, and ties the bag closed.

83. D: Pulse oximetry measures oxygenation but not ventilation. Patients who have 100% oxygenation could have respiratory acidosis from inadequate ventilation. Readings under 90% indicate significant hypoxemia. Bright lights interfere with the accuracy of the pulse oximeter, so cover the patient's hand bearing the oximeter with a drape or blanket. Methylene blue and other IV dyes may interfere with the performance of the pulse oximeter.

84. C: The *Sellick maneuver* involves pressing on the patient's cricoid cartilage with your index finger, or thumb and forefinger. The Sellick maneuver provides better visualization of the tracheal lumen and occludes the esophagus to prevent regurgitation.

85. A: Phlebothrombosis may result if blood flow to the patient's legs is obstructed. Shearing results from moving the patient improperly. Air embolism is an air bubble floating in the circulatory system. Bronchospasm may occur upon extubation, but is not a result of faulty positioning.

86. C: Improper positioning of the patient's arm (or arm board) may result in injury to the brachial plexus.

87. A: The nurse who is monitoring a sedated patient should have *no other responsibilities*. A second perioperative nurse should circulate, and a third nurse should "scrub in" to assist the surgeon.

88. C: The sections of the stomach are the cardia, fundus, corpus (body), and pylorus.

89. D: The functions of the stomach include the receipt and storage of ingested materials. The stomach digests these substances using gastric lipase, pepsinogen, hydrochloric acid, gastrin and

intrinsic factor, which aids in the absorption of vitamin B_{12}. Alcohol is absorbed in the stomach, but *most* other ingested substances are absorbed in the small intestine. Peristalsis mixes and moves the stomach contents, or *chyme*, into the duodenum.

90. B: *Bariatric surgery* is another term for a weight reduction procedure, such as gastric bypass (stomach stapling). Bariatric patients are morbidly obese, usually 40 kg above their normal weight, or have a BMI above 40. Their health, mobility, environmental access, and socialization have degraded, due to their size.

91. A: ERCP stands for endoscopic retrograde cholangiopancreatography. An ERCP permits the surgeon to directly visualize the patient's biliary tract, to assesses the liver, pancreas and spleen. The surgeon injects radiographic dye into the ductal system and obtains biopsies whenever indicated. Angiography refers to a cardiologist's x-ray evaluation of a blood vessel. PET scans (positron emission tomography) produce cross-section images, usually of the brain, which reveal metabolic processes to the radiologist. The MRI (magnetic resonance imaging) is a Medical Imaging test that provides highly detailed, three dimensional images.

92. B: The Veress needle is the portal for inserting CO_2 gas into the patient's abdomen in the closed technique of pneumoperitoneum. The Veress needle has a retractable cutting sheath, which the surgeon inserts through a small supraumbilical incision into the peritoneal cavity. CO_2 tubing attaches to the Veress needle for insufflation.

93. C: The insufflation of CO_2 begins at a rate of 1 to 2 L/min, with a *maximum pressure level of 15 mm/Hg*. Higher pressures could result in CO_2 diffusion into the bloodstream, with ensuing respiratory acidosis, bradycardia, blood pressure changes, and possibly lethal gas embolism.

94. D: Herniorrhaphy (hernia) repair is the most common general surgery performed in the USA.

95. C: AORN recommends the use of chlorhexidine gluconate (CHG) as a cleansing agent during the patient's preoperative shower. CHG significantly inhibits the growth of *Staphylococcus epidermis,* and Gram-positive and Gram-negative bacteria, and viruses. By reducing surface skin colonization, CHG subsequently decreases the postoperative incidence of infection. Dove soap has no antibacterial properties. Povidone iodine and alcohol are often used in the O.R. as skin preps, but are inappropriate for showering.

96. A: Reattach her urinary catheter bag to a lower section of the cart to permit gravity drainage. If you place the drainage bag on your patient's abdomen, the urine drains back into her bladder, increasing her discomfort and chances of a urinary tract infection. Clamping the catheter and detaching it from the drainage tubing during transport would be time-consuming. Since it is imperative to move your patient to the Post Anesthesia Care Unit (PACU) as quickly as possible, your best choice is to hang her bag on a lower section of the cart.

97. C: The reverse Trendelenburg position is a version of the supine position, in which the patient's head rests higher than the feet.

98. B: An improperly placed, heavy, third trimester uterus pressurizes the vena cava and aorta, resulting in hypotension. Put a padded wedge under her right side to tilt her uterus laterally and alleviate pressure on the major vessels. Raising your patient's legs prevents venous pooling in her lower extremities, but does not relieve uterine pressure on her heart. A small pillow under her waist may improve her comfort in the supine position, but does not decrease the uterine burden.

Sequential compression stockings prevent blood from pooling in the legs, but have no effect on the pressure the uterus applies to the major blood vessels of the heart.

99. D: When placing the patient into the prone position, all your movements should be slow and gentle. A minimum of four people should work as a team to insure the patient's safety. The anesthesiologist supports the head and neck and maintains the position of the endotracheal tube. The second member of the perioperative team turns the patient onto his/her side on the stretcher. The third member, positioned on the opposite side of the operating table, 'catches' the patient while supporting the chest and abdomen. A fourth person turns the patient's legs in unison.

100. B: At least two people are necessary to transfer your patient from the stretcher to the operating table. Lock the wheels of the stretcher *and* operating table prior to moving your patient. Never assume the cleaner remembered to lock the operating table after disinfecting it; ensure the O.R. table will not roll. The stretcher should be the *same* level as the operating table prior to transferring your patient, not higher.

101. C: Electric clipping is the preferred method for removing hair from a surgical site. A razor blade may nick the area and increase the chances of infection. Hot wax pulls the hair and may result in inflammation of the area.

102. B: Shaving the patient in the O.R. could result in airborne hair contamination of the sterile fields. The Holding Area, where the patient awaits surgery, is the preferred location for the preoperative shave.

103. D: Both the circulating nurse and the scrub nurse *must* witness the sponge count. Quickly count with the scrub nurse, and then relay the message.

104. B: Begin counting with the sponges that are on the surgical field, sponge sticks, Mayo stand, and then the back table. The circulating nurse watches and confirms the count with the scrub nurse, completing the count with the soiled sponges. The final number must be the same as the number of sponges opened for the case.

105. A: If the sponge count is incorrect, inform the surgeon and anesthesiologist immediately. The patient may need to remain under anesthesia until an abdominal x-ray determines if the sponge is still inside the wound.

106. D: Assess the patient's skin prior to placement of the dispersive electrode. Scar tissue, excessive adipose tissue, metal prosthetic implants, bony prominences, pacemakers, and automatic cardiac defibrillators require special placement of the dispersive electrode.

107. A: Dispersive electrode pads are *not* interchangeable. Call for one that matches the machine, and if unavailable, exchange the machine for one that matches the pad. A hand-held cauterizer is suitable for minor cases, but is inappropriate for major surgeries. The dispersive electrode is useless if not attached to the correct generator.

108. B: *Cutting-point* needles have a razor-sharp tip for easily penetrating tough tissues, such as skin or tendon. Taper-point needles are appropriate for soft tissue, such as intestine or peritoneum. Blunt-tip needles are suitable for friable tissue, such as liver or kidney. "Saber-tip" is a misnomer.

109. B: The single lumen, rubber or silicone, Penrose drain is the most common *passive* drain. The Jackson-Pratt and Hemovac are *active* drains, in which the reservoir collapses to create negative pressure, directing the drainage into the reservoir. *Sump drains* are double-lumened and may attach to an external suction machine.

110. D: There are other closed drains that prevent wound contamination, such as the Stryker Constavac. Neither JP nor Hemovac attach to external suction, lie flat, nor contain double-lumens. JP drains are used to remove small amounts of pus, infectious fluid, and blood. The larger reservoir attached to Hemovac drain allows for accurate measurement of drainage, so it can be retained and reinfused to minimize the patient's blood loss.

111. B: The anesthesiologist (or nurse anesthetist) checks for proper placement of the endotracheal tube by listening to both lungs for breath sounds, observing fog in the endotracheal tube, and watching the end-tidal monitor for CO_2. Inspection of the oral cavity does not allow enough airway exposure for the anesthesiologist to determine the position of the endotracheal tube in the trachea.

112. D: During intubation, the perioperative nurse can: Pull outwardly on the corner of the patient's mouth to enhance visualization of the vocal chords; hold the endotracheal tube for easy access by the anesthetist; apply pressure (the Sellick maneuver) to the cricoid cartilage to enhance chord exposure: and provide a 10 mL syringe for inflation of the endotracheal tube cuff.

113. D: The surgical patient who ingested food or liquid within 8 hours of surgery requires special precautions to prevent potentially fatal aspiration of vomitus. Be prepared in case your patient regurgitates his stomach contents while under anesthesia. Gather a nasogastric tube, an emesis basin, a suction catheter or tip, and a clean towel. Sterilization is unnecessary. The Sellick maneuver blocks the esophagus and helps prevent aspiration.

114. C: Nitrous oxide is "laughing gas", a sweet-smelling, analgesic gas that rapidly produces mild euphoria and relaxation. It is a *supplement,* used in combination with stronger inhaled anesthetics to improve their action. Nitrous oxide is not a stand-alone anesthetic.

115. B: The anesthesia machine has a scavenger system, which connects to a suction line.

116. D: Frequent, prolonged exposure to anesthetic gases in the O.R. presents a serious health threat to perioperative staff. Beware of dizziness, nausea, headaches, fatigue, drowsiness, and decreased mental acuity in yourself or your teammates.

117. D: Exposure to anesthetic agents may cause miscarriages, reduced fertility, and liver, renal, and neurological diseases.

118. A: A Bier Block involves the intravenous injection of an anesthetic agent (usually Lidocaine) into the vein of an extremity bound by two tourniquets, or a double cuffed tourniquet. Prior to inflating the tourniquets, the nurse wraps the elevated extremity with the Esmarch bandage to enhance the blood drainage. The surgeon or anesthetist injects the anesthetic agent.

119. D: Passing instruments to the surgeon during surgery is the responsibility of the scrub nurse.

120. B: As the circulating perioperative nurse, you relay updates from the surgeon to the patient's family via telephone to the Waiting Room. (Often, a hospital volunteer screens your call to ensure

you are speaking with the correct person.) Your first obligation is to the patient, but you should keep the family informed. Leaving the O.R. to go to the Waiting Room is unnecessary.

121. A: The Joint Commission instituted a standardized approach to "hand-off" communications between perioperative personnel. The Holding Area nurse must provide *appropriate* information to the perioperative circulating nurse, which includes discussion of the proper surgical site, but is not limited to it.

122. D: The scrub nurse should leave these items on the back table until there is time to open and count them with the circulating nurse. Pass the surgeon the next instrument, then open and count the items.

123. B: The circulating nurse and the scrub nurse, who perform the counts, co-sign the *Perioperative Report.*

124. B: Tourniquet use can cause necrosis that may require amputation later. The information recorded regarding the tourniquet include: An assessment of the skin that will lie under the cuff, prior to its application; cuff location; type of material used under the cuff for skin protection; cuff pressure; calibration; time of inflation and deflation; identification, serial number and model of equipment used; name of the person applying the cuff; and an assessment of the entire extremity after use of the tourniquet.

125. A: The perioperative nurse does *not* record the amount of prep solution used.

126. D: The perioperative nurse who monitors a patient receiving local anesthetic should note the: Skin color and condition; mental status; amount of anesthetic administered; and vital signs (B/P, pulse rate and rhythm, respiration rate); and O_2 saturation. It is unnecessary to record the location of each injection.

127. B: The patient who receives local anesthetic may have a *toxic reaction* from rapid absorption by the circulatory system. Signs and symptoms of a toxic reaction, from mild to severe, are: Restlessness; dizziness; visual and auditory disturbances; tremors; convulsions; unconsciousness; apnea; and cardiac arrest.

128. D: Inform the surgeon of the signs and symptoms the patient is experiencing. Establish and maintain an airway and administer oxygen. Give sedation as ordered by the surgeon. Call the anesthesiologist for assistance, if necessary. Ensure the crash cart (resuscitation equipment) is in the room. Narcan is a drug used to counter the action of narcotics, not local anesthetics.

129. A: Assess your patient's skin both prior to and after surgery. Note the type of equipment used for positioning, such as stirrups for lithotomy position, placement of the extremities, and special precautions used to protect the eyes. Record any changes in the patient's position, the location of the safety strap, and the name of the person who positioned the patient. The height of the operating table and Mayo stand, and the number of staff assisting the surgeon do not affect the patient's position. If the table is elevated during the procedure, check the Mayo stand to ensure it does not rest directly on the patient.

130. D: The hand-off report includes: Patient demographics (name, age, and sex); type of anesthesia (local, general, regional, epidural, or spinal); anesthetic agent used; estimated blood

loss; intraoperative medications; fluid and blood administered; urinary output; lab results; chronic and acute history; drug allergies; problems and concerns; desired outcomes; and a discharge plan.

131. D: The scrub nurse must label all medications on the sterile field with either pre-printed labels or plain sterile labels with a sterile marker. The use of different containers helps identify the medication from a distance, but the container must have the name of the drug printed on it as a fail-safe.

132. A: When the surgeon gives a verbal order for medication during surgery, written confirmation of the drug and dosage is the preferred method for *verifying* the order. The surgeon, not the scrub nurse, is the person who substantiates medication and dosage. The perioperative nurse must check the patient's record for allergies prior to administering any medication, but this is not part of the verification process. A newly ordered medication during the surgery is not entered in the patient's record until the surgeon updates it, following the procedure.

133. C: The GI surgery patient should *avoid* carbonated beverages for three to four weeks to prevent painful gas bloating.

134. D: Discharge instructions include: Medication directions; pain management; wound care; signs and symptoms of infection and other complications; the surgeon's phone number; date to schedule a follow-up appointment; and any education specific to the surgery (e.g., a dialysis overview for a graft recipient). Itching and prickly sensations around the incision site are common during the healing process.

135. C: Any postoperative patient who received general anesthetic could develop a persistent cough. The *best* advice is for the patient to inform her physician. Your conversation may include questions regarding her temperature, and instructions for splinting and postural drainage. However, the patient needs to inform the physician in case she needs further treatment, such as chest physiotherapy, or prescriptions, such as antibiotics.

136. B: When the patient has to *"teach back"* (explain the instructions back to you), it allows you to evaluate his/her understanding of the discharge instructions. Correct any areas of misunderstanding. A written instruction booklet supports the verbal information you provided.

137. C: The GI patient should inform the physician about any of these signs and symptoms, but the increase in abdominal swelling or pain is especially important following surgery on the liver, biliary tract, pancreas or spleen.

138. D: Surgical patients who are most likely to contract MRSA include: High-risk patients with underlying diseases; those with prolonged hospitalizations; patients from Intensive Care Units; patients who have had previous antimicrobial therapy; and those who were exposed to other MRSA patients.

139. B: Steam sterilization is the oldest, safest, cheapest, and best understood method. Ethylene oxide is highly explosive, carcinogenic, toxic, and flammable. Dry heat takes two hours, so it is only appropriate for materials that cannot tolerate other methods of sterilization, such as powders, grease, anhydrous oils, and some glassware. Low-temperature hydrogen peroxide plasma is replacing ethylene oxide, but *Geobacillus stearothermophilus* spores may survive peroxidation.

140. D: Flash sterilization containers are not for the storage of sterile items. A single wrapper is appropriate for specialized instruments, if the manufacturer's instructions for the sterilizer indicate this is an approved sterilizing technique. Flash sterilization requires little or no drying time.

141. A: A biological indicator (BI) is a strip, ampoule, or capsule that contains live, highly resistant spores of a known type, to test the efficacy of a sterilizer. Chemical indicators contain a dye that changes color under certain conditions. Chemical indicators do not guarantee sterility, but determine that the parameters for sterilization have been met.

142. C: Steam sterilization may damage some plastics, melt some powders, and dilute some oils. Steam is readily available and leaves no toxic residue. Steam is economical and fast. Steam is appropriate for most surgical instruments and in-house packaging materials.

143. B: *Disinfection* is the process that kills pathogenic microorganisms through the application of a chemical germicide, with the exception of bacterial spores. Disinfection does not afford the same level of safety as sterilization. *Purification* means eliminating some unwanted contaminants, such as chlorine or lead. *Fumigation* is gas spray or bombs that eliminate pests, such as bed bugs.

144. D: *Prions* are infectious protein particles that are responsible for spongiform encephalopathies, such as CJD.

145. B: Prions are responsible for the transfer of CJD, an always fatal neurological disease. Prions resist routine sterilization and disinfection techniques. Protocols for sterilization of instruments following exposure to eye or neurological tissue of a CJD patient are evolving. The Center for Disease Control (CDC) and the World Health Organization (WHO) have the latest information on removing infectious prions.

146. B: Hair is a major source of *Staphylococcus*. The number of microorganisms found on hair correlates with the length and cleanliness of the hair.

147. D: Obesity increases the patient's risk of infection, due to the decreased blood supply in adipose tissue. Radiation therapy patients are immunocompromised and more prone to infection. Previous joint replacement should not increase the risk of infection for a patient's future surgeries.

148. B: The Joint Commission, Association of periOperative Registered Nurses (AORN), and World Health Organization (WHO) all recommend against wearing artificial nails. Chipped or broken artificial nails harbor significantly more microorganisms. *Well-maintained n*ail polish did not increase the microorganism count. No action was necessary.

149. B: The perioperative nurse should *never* attempt to sterilize a single-use item. The manufacturer must meet extremely stringent requirements for preparing a single-use item. If the nurse attempts to sterilize it, then the hospital assumes all liability. The nurse should phone Central Sterile Supply and send the item to them by porter. The CSS supervisor will decide if reprocessing complies with hospital policy. 2% alkaline glutaraldehyde can sterilize some items, but the immersion period is a minimum of 10 hours. The manufacturer would have to approve glutaraldehyde sterilization for this particular instrument. Inform the surgeon and anesthesiologist of the situation.

150. B: Once the pointed towel clip penetrates the drape, it becomes contaminated; removing it would involve pulling it back through the drape and contaminating the sterile field. The *best* option

is to re-clasp it. Ignoring the towel clip is inappropriate because it could fall and harm the patient with its sharp points. Removal of the towel clip by anyone would contaminate the sterile field.

151. C: Once the scrub nurse wears the gown, its cuffs, neckline, shoulder, and axillae are not sterile. The area below the waist and the back are not sterile. Sterile areas include the top edge of the cuffs to two inches above the elbow, and the front of the gown, from the chest to the level of the sterile field.

152. C: When dispensing a sterile item, open the flap furthest from you, proceed to the side flaps, and lastly remove the closest flap. After opening each flap, secure it with the other hand. Open heavy items on small tables or ring stands for the scrub nurse to retrieve.

153. D: After you remove the cap of NSS irrigation fluid and dispense it onto the sterile field, discard the remainder in the bottle. Recapping is inappropriate. The top of the bottle is considered contaminated, since drops may have encountered the outside of the bottle during the primary pouring.

154. D: Unscrubbed personnel should not walk between sterile fields. Unscrubbed personnel should keep a safe distance from sterile fields, and should face sterile fields.

155. B: A *Laminair* air flow systems are unidirectional ventilation systems, in which air passes through a high efficiency particulate air (HEPA) filter, which removes bacteria. This 'ultraclean' air circulates over the patient and then returns through a receiving air inlet. A Laminair system is often used in orthopedic surgery suites, where osteomyelitis is a danger.

156. D: Only smooth, nonporous, washable, easy to clean surfaces are appropriate for Operating Room use. Ridges harbor bacteria.

157. D: An increase in the number of people in the O.R. increases the quantity of microorganisms, and the possibility of a surgical site infection (SSI).

158. B: Dust and lint that carry microorganisms settle on horizontal surfaces.

159. C: A hospital-grade disinfectant that is approved by the EPA is appropriate for use in the O.R. *prior* to the first case of the day. Alcohol and high-level disinfectants used for instruments are inappropriate for use as cleansers in the O.R. because they are flammable. Formalin is a specimen preservative, but as a proven carcinogen, it is unsuitable as a cleanser. If the surgeon used cadaverous transplant material, or the patient had rapid-onset dementia, or the family history is suspicious for prion diseases, soak the instruments after surgery in a covered pan of 1N sodium hydroxide (NaOH) for 60 minutes, steam autoclave for 30 minutes at 121°C, AND follow up with routine sterilization. Check the CDC and WHO Web sites for the latest CJD decontamination techniques.

160. C: Schedule patients with airborne-transmitted diseases, such as tuberculosis (TB), to have surgery when personnel and patients are at a minimum (last case of the day).

161. D: Ophthalmic instruments are very delicate. Eye instruments must be hand-washed and their tips carefully examined for burrs.

162. A: The best method of transfer for dirty instruments is in a closed cart, to prevent inadvertent contamination of other hospital areas during transportation.

163. B: Once opened during surgery, special surgical instruments require reprocessing.

164. B: In the open technique, there is a greater chance of contamination.

165. A: A member of the surgical team who contaminates a glove must step away from the sterile field, wait for the circulating nurse to remove the contaminated glove, and finally re-glove.

166. B: Grasp the glove approximately 2" below your co-worker's wrist. Carefully remove it, taking care *not* to pull down the cuff. Once your coworker's hand went through the cuff, the cuff was contaminated.

167. D: The circulating nurse dons clean (unsterile) gloves and uses care not to cause further contamination.

168. A: AORN recommends the double-glove technique for invasive surgeries. Double-gloving decreases the number of perforations of the inner glove.

169. D: The anesthetized patient may experience vomiting, laryngospasms, or bronchospasms during extubation.

170. B: A large percentage of fires in the O.R. occur in the patient's facial area because of the oxygen-enriched atmosphere. Fires during abdominal surgeries may be due to ignition of the drape material by an active electrode.

171. B: Halon is the best fire extinguisher for the O.R. The halon extinguisher is lightweight, easy to use, and versatile. Although the label of a halon extinguisher states it is effective on Class B (flammable liquids and grease) and Class C (electrical) fires, it also works on Class A (wood, cloth, paper, and most plastics).

172. A: If a fiber-optic cord or connector detaches during use, the heat may result in a drape fire. Never place *uncoupled* cords on the patient's drapes. Remove fiber-optic headlights when the physician finishes with them, to eliminate the possibility of igniting surgical gowns or clothing.

173. C: *First and foremost,* remove the drapes to rescue the patient from the burning materials. Next, announce over the intercom system, "Code Red" and the location of fire. Turn off all room gases. Contain the fire. Extinguish it with water or saline from the back table, or with the halon fire extinguisher. When the fire is out, announce, "Code Red, all clear".

174. D: Pull the extinguisher's pin, aim the nozzle, squeeze the handle, and then sweep the stream at the base of the fire.

175. C: The circulating nurse should move any foot pedal that is not in use, so the surgeon does not inadvertently step on it. 100% oxygen is not a good choice for facial surgery because it is a fire hazard. A lower percentage of oxygen or air is appropriate for most patients. Air is in the yellow tank on an anesthesia machine. Shaving a man's beard or mustache is usually unnecessary; coating the hair with a water-based lubricant prevents fire. The electrosurgery pencil belongs in a holster when it is not in use; never rest it on the drape.

176. D: Place wet towels around the incision site when using a laser. The use of nonreflective instruments prevents the laser beam from reflecting onto unintended areas and possibly causing burns. The laser setting should be on "standby" when not in use.

177. A: Dantrolene sodium (Dantrium) is a skeletal muscle relaxant. Dantrium is the drug of choice for treating the rigid muscles and fever associated with malignant hyperthermia. If your patient experiences malignant hyperthermia, the anesthetist should discontinue the triggering anesthetic (usually halothane). Hyperventilate the patient with 100% O_2. Administer Dantrium by rapid IV push, 1 mg/kg. Do not mix Dantrium with D5W or normal saline. The doctor may order more Dantrium at three-minute intervals, for a total of 10 mg/kg, and add bromocriptine. If possible, terminate the surgery.

178. D: At least 36 vials of Dantrolene sodium (Dantrium) are necessary for a 175 pound patient. Reconstitute each vial with preservative-free sterile injectable water, and shake vigorously to achieve adequate mixing. Treat acidosis with sodium bicarbonate. A clearly written protocol sheet is very important. Have cold sterile saline available for wound irrigation, cold IV solution, ice or a cooling blanket, and equipment for cold gastric and rectal lavage. Since succinylcholine and halothane trigger malignant hyperthermia, replace the anesthesia machine with another one, if available. If another anesthesia machine is unavailable, change its circuits and carbon dioxide absorbent. Have a variety of Vacutainer blood vials ready.

179. B: The perioperative nurse should immediately inform the anesthesiologist and surgeon about the possibility of malignant hyperthermia. Muscle biopsy is a diagnostic test to rule out this life-threatening, inherited condition. Telling your patient that the fever was probably due to an infection is an assumption with no supporting evidence. Informing your patient that the anesthetist will monitor his body temperature is accurate, but if the patient has a history of malignant hyperthermia, it is imperative to get a proper diagnosis prior to administering anesthesia. His body temperature is more likely to drop as a response to the cool O.R., so the warm blanket may help prevent hypothermia.

180. B: Chemical manufacturers provide a safety data sheet (SDS, formerly MSDS) for each chemical they sell. The SDS describes the dangers of each chemical and first-aid measures in the event of exposure. If you cannot find the SDS, phone your Safety Officer.

181. D: Methyl methacrylate is an acrylic, cement-type compound used in some orthopedic and neurosurgery cases. The nurse removes his/her contact lenses to prevent eye damage from penetrating vapors. Wear a face shield and double gloves. Mix the chemicals under a fume hood or suction evacuation bowl. Ensure there are no sparks or open flames, as the liquid component is highly flammable. Pour the liquid (PMMA) into the powder, to minimize aerosolization. Polymerization will form the compound into a durable plastic.

182. C: The O.R. supervisor must have a blend of management, clinical, interpersonal, technological, and financial expertise.

183. A: Efficient turn-over of Operating Rooms between cases is a cost-saving technique. Skipping breaks is not cost-efficient. Perioperative personnel work in a high stress environment and benefit from rest periods. Scratched laser glasses could allow laser beams to damage the eyes. Sterile NSS, once poured, is contaminated.

184. D: Numerous factors influence surgical scheduling. Schedule infectious patients late in the day. The availability of specialty rooms, teams, and equipment are important. Surgeons usually have certain hours set aside for surgical cases. Coordinating with the surgeon's office is an important aspect of creating a schedule. The lunch schedule varies with the float nurses' availability changes, and as cases finish. Lunch breaks are an ongoing concern for the nurse who is coordinating the day's cases as they unfold.

185. B: Firstly, establish the requirements for the new drape materials. Secondly, contact multiple manufacturers and have their representatives set up product demonstrations. Thirdly, compare costs and quality from one manufacturer to the next, including thickness of the drape material and fire-resistance. Evaluate single drapes vs. combination packages with cost comparisons. Other considerations include ease of use, staff opinions of sample materials, and environmental impact from disposal.

186. D: The Nurse's Five Rights Of Delegation include the right task, right circumstances, right person, right communication, and right supervision.

187. A: The *Perioperative Patient-Focused Model* emphasizes the *outcome-driven* nature of perioperative patient care. The prevention of injury, reduction of risk, and implementation of a nursing care plan are parts of this overall plan.

188. A: Evidence-based practice is the systematic, meticulous process used to identify an issue, to gather and assess the best evidence to draft and employ a practice change and to evaluate the process. To find out more about evidence-based practice, visit the Centre for Health Evidence at http://www.cche.net/default.asp .

189. D: Performance improvement techniques encompass improvements in quality and effectiveness, based on moral and economical perspectives.

190. A: The sterile surgical team takes direction from the surgeon. The non-sterile team set up the non-sterile equipment, assist the anesthetist, and position the anesthetized patient.

191. D: The circulating nurse is the patient's advocate, who coordinates intraoperative patient care. The circulating nurse manages and implements activities outside the sterile field. The goal of the circulating nurse is to achieve desirable patient outcomes.

192. D: In addition to assisting the anesthetist, standing next to the patient during induction provides emotional support and prevents patient falls.

193. D: The nurse manager assigns scrub personnel based on their expertise. The staffing skill mix must be appropriate to the procedure and hospital policy. Seniority does not equate with expertise.

194. A: The physician's preference cards include the preferred sutures, special instruments or equipment, and types of dressing. The surgeon's phone number is not included. The physician's preference card does not contain each and every instrument the surgeon would use, since most specialties have pre-arranged trays that include common instruments. The surgeon does not decide on the staff; that is the prerogative of the nurse manager.

195. A: The temperature of the room is not recorded on the O.R. record.

196. D: The perioperative nurse exercises active listening, and offers the patient reassurance to alleviate anxiety. All surgery carries some risk. Telling the patient that there is nothing to fear is inappropriate.

197. D: The perioperative nurse monitors blood pressure, EKG, and oxygen saturation for the patient who receives local anesthetic. The nurse also ensures the crash cart (resuscitation equipment) stands ready nearby.

198. D: The circulating nurse and scrub nurse co-sign the sponge counts on the *Perioperative Report*.

199. A: Head injuries may occur when the overhead lights are positioned for surgery.

200. C: Occupational hazards in the nurse's workplace include: Needle sticks; slips and falls; head injuries; chemical, radiation, and anesthetic gas exposures; and back injuries. Occupational hazards lead many nurses to leave their profession. Nurses in the O.R. wear personal protective equipment (PPE) when exposed to infectious materials. Depending on the facility, most nurses have choices regarding their preferred hours of work. There are difficult people in every profession. Disagreeable surgeons are not a recognized reason for nurses leaving their profession.

Practice Test #2

Practice Questions

1. The nursing process is essential in developing a perioperative plan of care. This six-part process includes assessment, nursing diagnosis, identifying outcomes, implementation, evaluation, and
____.
    a. Benchmarking
    b. Planning
    c. Communicating
    d. Interventions

2. Which of the following best describes the purpose of informed consent?
    a. To prevent health information privacy violations
    b. To inform the patient of which physician will be performing the procedure
    c. To explain to the patient the type and purpose of the procedure as well as the risks, benefits, alternatives, and complications associated with it
    d. To alleviate the legal burden of a poor outcome

3. Who has the responsibility to obtain informed consent?
    a. Surgeon
    b. Circulating RN
    c. Primary MD
    d. Preoperative RN

4. Which of the following is the best method to prevent intraoperative patient burns when using an electrosurgical unit (ESU)?
    a. Leave the ESU pencil on the surgical drape in open view between uses
    b. Ensure adequate skin contact of the patient return electrode
    c. Place the patient return electrode over a previous surgical site
    d. Do not use any alcohol-based surgical preps in the operating room

5. Which of the following is an example of manual hemostasis?
    a. Laser
    b. Fibrin glue
    c. Sutures
    d. Electrosurgical unit (ESU)

6. Your patient is scheduled for an arteriovenous (AV) fistula creation. She is a 62-year-old female with Type 1 diabetes. Which potential complication should the circulating nurse be aware of intraoperatively?
    a. Infection
    b. Delayed wound healing
    c. Hypotension
    d. Hypertension

7. Which of the following is a common indication for surgery in the pediatric population?
   a. Congenital anomalies
   b. Prematurity
   c. Low birth weight
   d. Fetal alcohol syndrome

8. You are the circulating RN for an appendectomy on a three-year-old female. When transporting her to the operating room, you might expect her to demonstrate which behavior?
   a. Concerns for physical appearance after the surgery
   b. Crying for parents
   c. Pretends to be Wonder Woman
   d. Nonverbal sounds only

9. While performing a Nissen fundoplication, the surgeon asks you to place the bed in the reverse Trendelenburg position. Which of the following best describes this position?
   a. Dorsal recumbent
   b. Supine with the head of the bed lower than the feet
   c. Supine with the head of the bead higher than the feet
   d. Supine with the patient's legs elevated in stirrups

10. You are helping place a patient in the lateral position for a right thoracotomy surgery. You should be aware of the potential for which injury with this type of position?
    a. Lower back strain
    b. Pressure ulcers to the posterior skull
    c. Nerve damage to the extremities
    d. Skin tears on the buttocks

11. You are the postanesthesia care nurse caring for a pediatric trauma patient. The surgeon has ordered morphine sulfate (MS) for postoperative pain control. Which of the following is the most appropriate pediatric dosage?
    a. 0.1–0.2 mg/kg IV
    b. 0.1–0.2 mg/kg PO
    c. 1–2 mg/kg IV
    d. 0.5–1 mg/kg IM

12. Which of the following is a therapeutic effect specific to midazolam hydrochloride?
    a. Nausea and vomiting
    b. Respiratory depression
    c. Short-term and retrograde amnesia
    d. Pain control

13. Which of the following is a defect of tetralogy of Fallot?
    a. Stenosis of the aortic valve
    b. Stenosis of the pulmonary valve
    c. Hypertrophy of the left ventricle
    d. Displacement of the aorta to the left

14. In elderly patients, why would the perioperative nurses want to carefully monitor which medications the patient is given postoperatively?
  a. Drug tolerance can be very high in the elderly due to the large number of medications they may regularly take
  b. Elderly patients metabolize anesthesia medications very quickly and will require larger doses of pain medications for comfort
  c. Elderly patients have many more drug allergies
  d. Elderly patients are more prone to drug interactions because they have lower tolerance and excretion of medications

15. What is the difference between the semirestricted and restricted areas of the operating room department?
  a. In the semirestricted areas, you can wear street clothes, but in the restricted area, you must wear surgical scrubs
  b. Both areas require you to wear surgical scrubs, but in the restricted area you must wear a hair covering
  c. There is no semirestricted area in the operating room, just an unrestricted and restricted
  d. In both areas, you must wear scrubs and a hair cover, but in the restricted areas, you must also wear a surgical mask

16. The room temperature in the operating room suites must be maintained within a specific range. Which one of the following answers provides the correct temperature range?
  a. 68°–73° F
  b. 65°–70° F
  c. 55°–60° F
  d. 65°–75° F

17. You are recovering a postoperative total hip replacement patient. What Aldrete score would you give her if she is fully awake and moving all extremities, her blood pressure is being maintained at her preoperative state, but she is having difficulty breathing deeply, and her O2 saturation is 92% with 2L oxygen per nasal cannula?
  a. 10
  b. 6
  c. 8
  d. 9

18. You are scrubbing a total abdominal hysterectomy. In which areas are you considered sterile after you don your sterile gown and gloves?
  a. Everywhere covered by the gown
  b. Only your hands
  c. Chest to sterile field
  d. Front and back of gown, chest to waist

19. You are the circulating RN on a laparoscopic cholecystectomy, and you see the suction tip is extending off the edge of the sterile back table but has not fallen off. What should you do?
  a. Tell the scrub tech so she can move it back on the table before it falls
  b. Tell the scrub tech to discard the tip
  c. Nothing: as long as it's still on the table, it's still sterile
  d. Remove it from the back table yourself

20. Unsterile personnel, such as the circulating RN, should stay away from the sterile field to avoid contamination. Which of the following is the minimum distance an unsterile person should remain from the sterile field?

    a. 15 in.

    b. 6 in.

    c. 12 cm

    d. 1 ft.

21. You are the circulating RN and are unwrapping a sterile endoscope for the sterile scrub tech. Which of the following best describes the technique used when unwrapping a sterile instrument as an unsterile person?

    a. Open the top flap away from you, then the sides, and then the bottom, being careful not to let the flaps touch each other so the edges do not contaminate each other

    b. Open the top flap away from you, then the sides, and then the bottom, securing each flap so they cover your unsterile hand and do not contaminate the sterile field or instrument

    c. The scrub tech should open sterile items because she is already sterile

    d. No real method exists as long as you do not touch the sterile item

22. You are working in the sterile processing department (SPD). The steam sterilizer has finished its cycle. What should you do with these sterile items?

    a. Unload them and leave them to dry on a table for 30 minutes

    b. Open the door of the sterilizer, and leave the products inside to dry for 15 to 60 minutes

    c. Unload the items and up them away immediately, so there is no inadvertent contamination

    d. Place the sterilizer on the drying cycle

23. You are scrubbing an exploratory laparotomy. You place an instrument magnet pad on the sterile field to prevent the instruments from falling. Which of the following should you not place on the instrument magnet?

    a. Needle holder

    b. Tenaculum clamp

    c. Mayo scissor

    d. Poole suction tip

24. For which piece of the following equipment should you place a return electrode on the patient?

    a. Electrosurgical unit (ESU)

    b. Greenlight laser

    c. Ultrasonic dissector

    d. Flexible endoscope

25. There are three types of blood loss replacements used in the perioperative setting. Autotransfusion is an example of which one of the following?

    a. Allogenous blood transfusion

    b. Autologous blood transfusion

    c. Blood product substitution

    d. Blood volume expander

26. You are the scrub RN for a surgery using a laser. Which of the following personnel safety precautions is most appropriate?
    a. Wearing a mask with a splash shield
    b. Wearing safety goggles with the correct optical density for the laser being used
    c. Wearing a N-95 mask
    d. Wearing latex-free gloves

27. Which of the following would be an appropriate environmental safety precaution when performing procedures utilizing lasers?
    a. Placing warning signs outside the OR suite that a laser is being used
    b. Removing all fluids from the surgical area so they do not spill on the laser
    c. Keeping the laser armed at all times so it is ready when needed
    d. Keeping an ABC-type fire extinguisher in the room

28. What does NPO stand for in relation to the perioperative setting?
    a. Nil per os
    b. Next patient operation
    c. New post operation
    d. Nil per ojos

29. In order to ensure proper functioning of the anesthesia monitoring equipment, patients should be informed to remove which of the following before surgery?
    a. Jewelry
    b. Glasses
    c. Dentures
    d. Nail polish and acrylic nails

30. You are the preoperative RN preparing to interview your patient for the preoperative assessment for her surgery. After washing your hands and introducing yourself to her, what is the first thing you should do?
    a. Check that the patient's surgical consent is correct and complete
    b. Review the surgeon's history and physical for past surgeries that could affect your plan of care
    c. Properly identify the patient by name and date of birth
    d. Check for medication allergies

31. During your preoperative assessment, your patient tells you she takes ginkgo biloba to help with her memory. What should you do?
    a. Nothing, this is an herbal and has no effect on the surgery
    b. Cancel the surgery because this medication has severe adverse reactions with the anesthetic agents
    c. Be sure this medication is added to her home medication list, and verify that the surgeon and anesthesia care provider are aware she takes it
    d. Ask the physician for a stat electrocardiogram (EKG), because this herbal can cause cardiac arrhythmias

32. The American Society of Anesthesiologists (ASA) status III would apply to which of the following patients?
    a. Healthy patient
    b. Mild systemic disease
    c. Brain death
    d. Severe systemic disease

33. Why should the surgical patient without a Foley catheter be encouraged to void in the preoperative area, if possible?
    a. To check for pregnancy
    b. To run a stat urinalysis
    c. To prevent bladder distention
    d. To prevent urinary tract infection

34. Mrs. Smith is scheduled for an endovascular procedure. She is allergic to shellfish. Which of the following could be affected by this allergy?
    a. Antibiotic choice
    b. Use of latex products
    c. Use of contrast media
    d. Administration of propofol

35. Many medications are administered during the perioperative phase. The five "rights" of safe medication administration include right patient, drug, dose, route, and which of the following?
    a. Method
    b. Physician
    c. Time
    d. Order

36. Your patient is going into respiratory arrest after a 2 mg dose of Versed. Which of the following medications would be the most appropriate to reverse the effects of this medication?
    a. Romazicon
    b. Narcan
    c. Benadryl
    d. Epinephrine

37. There have been a lot of reports in the media regarding intraoperative awareness. Which of the following pieces of equipment can help the anesthesia care provider prevent this complication?
    a. Electroencephalogram (EEG)
    b. Electrocardiogram (EKG)
    c. Bispectral index (BIS) monitoring
    d. Pulse oximetry

38. What does a reading of 100 on the BIS monitor means?
    a. The patient is fully awake
    b. The patient is highly sedated
    c. The patient is clinically brain dead
    d. The BIS monitoring machine is malfunctioning

39. You are the circulating RN caring for a patient receiving a carpal tunnel release under a brachial nerve block. When you document the type of anesthesia, you should list which of the following?

a. General anesthesia
b. Epidural anesthesia
c. Regional anesthesia
d. Monitored anesthesia care

40. Which of the following is one of the most commonly used medications for epidural anesthesia?
    a. Meperidine
    b. Bacitracin
    c. Bupivacaine
    d. Succinylcholine

41. The anesthesia care provider has informed you she will be performing a Bier block on your patient. Which piece of equipment would be necessary to perform this procedure?
    a. Electrosurgical unit (ESU)
    b. Single-cuff tourniquet
    c. Double-cuff tourniquet
    d. BIS monitor

42. As the circulating RN caring for a patient receiving a Bier block, which of the following is a very important consideration at the conclusion of the procedure with this type of anesthesia?
    a. Once the tourniquet is released, the surgical site will have a large amount of drainage
    b. These patients have a great deal of pain once the tourniquet is released
    c. There are no different concerns with Bier blocks than any other anesthesia
    d. The tourniquet should be released slowly to prevent a bolus of medication into the patient

43. It is imperative for the surgical team to keep track of sponges and instruments used during the surgery so that items are not inadvertently left in a patient. Which three positions and in which order should closing counts be performed?
    a. Field, floor (off the sterile field), back table
    b. Back table, floor, field
    c. Initial, baseline, final
    d. Field, back table, floor

44. What should the circulating RN do while the anesthesia care provider is intubating the patient during general anesthesia?
    a. Stay by the head of the bed and assist as needed
    b. Leave the room to get supplies
    c. Help the scrub nurse count instruments
    d. Start her charting

45. You are the circulating RN assisting the anesthesia care provider with a general anesthesia induction on a patient with a history of gastroesophageal reflux disease (GERD). The anesthesia care provider asks you to perform cricoid pressure. What is the purpose of cricoid pressure?
    a. To keep the patient's neck stable during tube placement
    b. To open the esophagus and allow air to enter the stomach to prevent gastric acid regurgitation
    c. To prevent aspiration of gastric contents while the patient does not have a proper gag reflex
    d. To hide the vocal cords because they are not a needed landmark to intubate

46. You the circulating RN for a patient who is having a vaginal hysterectomy. After assisting the anesthesia care provider, you need to place the patient's legs in stirrups. You should always check with the anesthesia care provider to be sure it is safe to position the patient. Which of the following provides the best answer of why the patient should not be moved until the anesthesia provider says it is safe?
   a. To give the anesthesia provider time to connect the vital sign monitors
   b. Because the patient may fall off the OR table if you position without the other providers' awareness
   c. To prevent accidental extubation
   d. Because the anesthesia provider may still need to place invasive lines

47. As a circulating RN you should be aware of possible complications that may occur during the procedure. Which of the following is the most common potential complication of femoropopliteal (fem-pop) bypass surgery?
   a. Renal damage from the on-table angiograms
   b. Nerve damage
   c. Operative leg swelling
   d. Femoral artery aneurysm

48. Why is spinal cord damage an operative risk with thoracic aortic aneurysm repair?
   a. Because the spinal cord may be cut in the procedure
   b. Because the spinal cord may experience ischemia if the cross-clamp time is excessive
   c. Because these patients are at high risk of stroke
   d. Because these patients often have already had spine surgery

49. You are the postanesthesia care RN recovering a new postoperative open appendectomy patient. Which of the following is the most appropriate in regards to how often should you normally monitor vital signs in the first postoperative hour in the PACU?
   a. Once
   b. Every 45 minutes
   c. Every 5 minutes
   d. Every 30 minutes

50. You are recovering a cesarean section patient in the PACU. If the patient received a regional anesthetic in the operating room, such as a spinal, which of the following would be the most important for the PACU nurse to monitor?
   a. The patient's dermatome levels
   b. The patient's height and weight
   c. The patient's input and output
   d. The patient's level of consciousness

Questions 51 - 53 refer to the following vignette:
   An 84-year-old lady with an ASA score of 4 and many comorbidities is scheduled for a new pacemaker placement. She is complaining of being cold and is beginning to shiver.

51. It is important as the perioperative nurse caring for this patient to be aware that shivering may lead to which of the following?
   a. Cardiac ischemia
   b. Respiratory depression

c. Hemorrhage

d. Stroke

52. Which is the most effective method to deal with this patient's hypothermia in the OR suite?

a. Warmed IV fluids

b. A forced-air warming blanket

c. It is not necessary to warm the patient because she will be asleep soon.

d. Regular blankets that have not been warmed

53. Once the pacemaker procedure is finished, this patient is moved to the PACU area to recover from her anesthesia. As the PACU RN, you should anticipate which of the following routine orders for this patient?

a. Ultrasound of pedal pulses

b. Blood transfusion

c. Chest X ray

d. Additional intravenous line placements

54. You have finished scrubbing a surgery and are breaking down your sterile field. What do you do with your surgical sharps, such as suture needles?

a. Place them in a biohazard bag

b. Place them in a puncture-proof sharps container

c. Place them in a puncture-proof box to be resterilized

d. Place them in a regular trash bag

55. As the circulating RN, you should verify that the anesthesia provider has given preoperative antibiotics as ordered by the surgeon. In what time frame should these be given for a patient who is not already on routine antibiotics?

a. 24 hours before the surgical incision

b. 6 hours before the surgical incision

c. 1 hour before the surgical incision

d. 2 days after the surgery

56. Traffic into the OR suite should be limited. No unneeded personnel should be in the suite, and the staff should try to limit trips in and out of the room. What is the purpose of this traffic control?

a. It is one of several methods to limit microbes in the OR

b. It is a security measure that is only used in emergency situations

c. It keeps distractions to the team to a minimum

d. Limitation of additional personnel in the OR suite is a safety measure the hospital institutes so there is less chance of injuries

57. You are the circulating RN, and your patient is having an exploratory laparotomy in the supine position. When the patient is in a supine position with arms extended, how should his palms be placed?

a. They should face up (supination)

b. They should face down (pronation)

c. Positioning the hands is not important

d. They should be placed lateral facing toward the body

58. How should a pregnant patient in the supine position be positioned differently than a nonpregnant patient?

a. She should have a wedge placed under her left side
b. She should have a pillow placed under her lower back
c. She should have a wedge placed under her right side
d. She should have a shoulder roll placed under her neck

59. You are the circulating RN for an obese patient that needs to be placed in a right lateral position. Multiple staff members and the surgeon come in to help with proper positioning. Which of the following is the most important regarding documentation of positioning?
    a. The number of people required to properly position
    b. Names of all team members and physicians involved with positioning the patient
    c. Preoperative skin condition
    d. Any invasive lines or drains that the patient came into the OR with

60. Operating room bed mattresses are made of different materials, much like a bed in your residence. In reference to prevention of pressure ulcers, which of the following is an effective OR table mattress material?
    a. Foam
    b. Synthetic down
    c. Springs
    d. Gel

61. You know your patient, who is a smoker, has additional healthcare risks to take in account when planning his plan of care. Compared to the other patients, what are smokers' risks for developing pressure ulcers during a long surgical procedure?
    a. They are at higher risk for pressure ulcer formation
    b. They are at lower risk for pressure ulcer formation
    c. They are at the same risk for pressure ulcer formation
    d. They are not at any risk for pressure ulcers because smoking causes vasodilatation

62. One of the factors in determining a patient's acuity score is the length of the surgery time. After how many hours in the same position is the patient's injury risk increased?
    a. 1 hour
    b. 2 hours
    c. 3 hours
    d. 0.5 hours

63. You are preparing to scrub for a surgery. Which of the following is the best place for you to open your sterile gown and gloves so you can don them after your surgical scrub?
    a. On the sterile back table
    b. On a separate sterile surface other than the back table
    c. On the sterile field
    d. Outside the OR suite

64. In which of the following scenarios would it be acceptable for the scrub nurse to open her sterile gown and gloves on the sterile back table?
    a. It is never recommended to do this
    b. When there is a sterile member, such as the scrub nurse she is relieving, to gown and glove her
    c. When there is no other surface available
    d. Once the patient has been draped, but the skin incision has not yet been made

65. How does the phrase "event-related" apply to supplies in the operating room?
    a. Package integrity
    b. Surgical time
    c. Surgical type
    d. Bulk sales from vendors

66. When placing sterile drapes around the surgical site to create the sterile field, how should the drapes be held?
    a. Higher than the OR table and placed from the surgical site outward
    b. Higher than the OR table and placed from the outside in toward the surgical site
    c. Under the OR table and brought around the patient
    d. It does not matter as long as you do not touch anything nonsterile with the sterile drapes

67. If a nonsterile equipment item is to be used in the sterile field, such as a C-arm device or ultrasound Doppler, what is the best way to use it and protect the surgical wound?
    a. The equipment should be covered with a sterile drape
    b. It does not need to be draped because the field is already sterile
    c. No special handling is required because is not a contamination risk
    d. Simply cover the surgical site with a sterile towel when using the nonsterile equipment

68. When is it ok to use an expired item?
    a. If it is an emergency
    b. If no replacement items are available
    c. Expiration dates are just a guide not a set-in-stone rule. As long as the item is intact, it is always ok to use these items
    d. You should never use an expired item

69. You are the circulating RN, and you are pouring sterile normal saline on the back field. You do not use all of the fluid in the container. Is it ok to recap the bottle and use the rest of the solution later on the field?
    a. Yes
    b. No
    c. Sometimes, if you kept the can sterile
    d. It does not matter, because sterile solutions are not used in the OR

70. Once the patient is brought into the surgical suite and transferred from her gurney to the OR table, what should you do?
    a. A safety strap is placed over her thighs
    b. A staff member stays and holds her in place
    c. No safety strap is necessary because the patient is not sedated
    d. A safety strap is placed across the chest

71. What is the minimum number of staff members needed to safely transfer a patient who can assist?
    a. 1
    b. 2
    c. 3
    d. 4

72. You are circulating a trauma and you request packed red blood cells (PRBCs) to give to the patient in the OR suite. Unless you keep the blood units in a cooler, how long can the units be out of the refrigerator before they cannot be returned to blood bank?
    a. 10 minutes
    b. 30 minutes
    c. 1 hour
    d. 15 minutes

73. You are transfusing a patient in the PACU, and you suspect an adverse blood reaction. What is the first thing you should do?
    a. Rush the blood in to prevent hypovolemia from the impending shock
    b. Send the unused blood to the blood bank
    c. Stop the transfusion
    d. Administer a bolus of normal saline

74. Whenever blood products are given to a patient, the correct information must be verified. Who can check blood products in the OR?
    a. Anyone
    b. Only the surgeon and anesthesia care provider
    c. Any two licensed professionals
    d. Only the blood bank staff

75. You are circulating a trauma. Your patient was in a motor vehicle accident, and, unfortunately, he does not survive. Which outside department should the circulating nurse call to report the patient's death?
    a. Fire department
    b. Media
    c. Coroner's office
    d. Funeral home

76. The coroner has released your deceased patient, and you are preparing to transfer him to the morgue. Where should the circulating nurse place the patient's identification tags before transport?
    a. On the patient and on the chart, anywhere visible
    b. On the patient and the shroud
    c. Only one tag is needed on the gurney transporting the patient.
    d. As long as the patient has an identification armband, he does not need additional identification tags.

77. After the surgical scrub, if the scrub nurse is not using an alcohol-based scrub product, she will need to dry her hands. Which of the following is the best method to pick up the sterile towel?
    a. Unfold it with both hands
    b. By the corner, with one hand
    c. In the middle, with one hand
    d. It does not matter how she picks up the towel

78. Now that the scrub nurse has properly grasped the sterile towel, which of the following best describes in which direction should she dry her hands and arms?
    a. From the fingers upward toward the elbow, without going backward
    b. From the upper arm down to the fingers
    c. From the fingers upward toward the elbow and then back down

d. Upward from one hand to the other, and then both forearms

79. In regard to marking a surgical site when a side is specified, which of the following persons should mark the surgical site?
    a. The patient
    b. The preoperative RN
    c. The circulating RN
    d. The surgeon

80. You will be circulating a total knee replacement. You ask the surgeon to mark the site. Which of the following should be used to mark the surgical site?
    a. A permanent skin marker
    b. A pen
    c. Any marker is appropriate, as long as the site is marked
    d. It is not necessary to mark the site, as long as you have radiographs available

81. When the surgeon is marking a surgical site, which of the following methods is most appropriate?
    a. Placing an X on the surgical site
    b. Writing YES on the surgical site
    c. Writing NO on the nonsurgical site
    d. Placing his initials on the surgical site

82. In addition to surgical site marking, a "time out" is performed by the surgical team to ensure the right patient and planned procedure is agreed upon. When should this process take place?
    a. In the preoperative holding area
    b. Immediately before the procedure
    c. After the surgeon makes the incision
    d. Prior to draping the patient

83. You are circulating a surgery, and the planned position is prone. Which of the following would be appropriate equipment needed for this type of positioning?
    a. Chest rolls/bolsters
    b. Stirrups
    c. Footboard
    d. Vacuum-assisted positioning device (beanbag)

84. The Kraske position is also known as which of the following?
    a. Lithotomy
    b. Supine
    c. Jackknife
    d. Lateral

85. The Kraske, or jackknife, position would be appropriate for which of the following procedures?
    a. Total vaginal hysterectomy
    b. Total abdominal hysterectomy
    c. Rectal surgery
    d. Thyroidectomy

86. What is the primary purpose of the surgical skin prep?
    a. To sterilize the surgical site
    b. To eliminate skin flora
    c. To reduce skin flora by chemically decontaminating the site
    d. To degrease the skin

87. When performing a skin prep, the circulating nurse must be aware of which body parts are considered contaminated in relation the surgical site so she will know how to prep. Which of the following body parts is considered contaminated and should be prepped first if it is included in the surgical field?
    a. Foot
    b. Breast
    c. Hand
    d. Umbilicus

88. You are preparing to perform a skin prep on a patient who is having an autologous skin graft placed over a debrided ulcer site on her right foot. The surgeon has informed you that the donor site will be the patient's left thigh. Which of the following best describes how you should perform the surgical skin prep for this patient?
    a. You should use one prep set, prepping the recipient site and then the donor site
    b. You need to prep the recipient site but not the donor site, because you are only removing skin from that area
    c. You should first prep the donor site using a colorless prep, and then prep the recipient site
    d. You should first prep the recipient site using a colorless prep, and then prep the donor site

89. Which of the following is an example of an antiseptic solution often found as an ingredient in surgical skin preps?
    a. Chlorhexidine gluconate
    b. Acetone
    c. Water
    d. ChloraPrep

90. An ever-present risk when giving general anesthesia is triggering a malignant hyperthermia (MH) incident. What is the test used to determine MH susceptibility?
    a. Myoglobin urine test
    b. Allergy testing
    c. Caffeine-halothane contracture test
    d. Ab1 testing

91. The medication of choice to treat malignant hyperthermia is which of the following?
    a. Dantrolene
    b. Propofol
    c. Succinylcholine
    d. Lasix

92. You are recovering a patient in the PACU who had a malignant hyperthermia event in the operating room. How long after the original MH episode must the patient receive dantrolene intravenously?
    a. 1–2 hours
    b. 24–72 hours
    c. 8–12 hours
    d. 5 days

93. What is the recommended dose range for IV dantrolene?
    a. 1.5 mg/kg initially, up to 15 mg/kg
    b. 0.25 mg/kg initially, up to 10 mg/kg
    c. 1.5 mg/lb initially, up to 50 mg/lb
    d. 2.5 mg/kg initially, up to 10 mg/kg

94. You are the primary circulator in the operating room for a patient in a MH crisis. Which of the following IV solutions is contraindicated during this time?
    a. Lactated Ringer's (LR)
    b. Normal saline (NS)
    c. Dextrose (D5)
    d. Potassium chloride (KCL)

95. Which of the following is a discharge criterion of Phase II but not Phase I of the postanesthesia care unit (PACU)?
    a. Airway patency
    b. Pain level
    c. Level of consciousness
    d. Gag reflex

96. Which of the following is a discharge assessment area in Phase I of PACU but not in Phase II?
    a. Airway patency
    b. Nausea level
    c. Level of consciousness
    d. Motor and sensory function

97. You are the scrub RN in the operating room. The surgeon asks for a fenestrated drape. Which of the following gives the best definition of what a fenestrated drape is?
    a. A drape with openings
    b. A folded towel
    c. Any folded drape
    d. An adhesive clear drape

98. Laparoscopic surgeries, such as laparoscopic cholecystectomy, require gas to be infused in the abdomen. The following three questions refer to this type of surgery. What type of gas is used?
    a. Argon
    b. Carbon dioxide
    c. Carbon monoxide
    d. Nitrogen

99. Which of the following is the recommended abdominal pressure during laparoscopic cases?
    a. 30–45mm Hg

b. 12–15mm Hg

c. 5–10mm Hg

d. 12–15mL

100. What is the purpose of introducing gas into the abdomen during laparoscopic surgeries?

    a. Better visualization of internal structures

    b. Control bleeding

    c. Compress internal organs

    d. To give the surgeon a method to insert instruments into abdomen

101. Some surgeries, especially orthopedic procedures on extremities, use pneumatic tourniquets to control intraoperative bleeding. The following three questions refer to the use of this device in the operating room. Which of the following personnel determines the pressure setting on the tourniquet?

    a. Surgeon

    b. Circulating RN

    c. Scrub RN

    d. Assistant

102. Although pressure settings may be adjusted as needed, what is the normal recommended range for tourniquet pressure on upper extremities?

    a. 30–70mm Hg below systolic blood pressure

    b. 30–70mL

    c. 30–70mm Hg above systolic blood pressure

    d. 30–70mm Hg above diastolic blood pressure

103. In order to prevent damage to the limb being constricted by a pneumatic tourniquet, it is vital to monitor the time the tourniquet has been inflated. After what amount of time should the limb be evaluated and the tourniquet be briefly deflated?

    a. 30-minute intervals

    b. 2-hour intervals

    c. 15 minutes

    d. 1 hour

104. Which of the following sutures should not be used in an infected surgical site?

    a. Gut

    b. Prolene

    c. Nylon

    d. Vicryl

105. Which of the following is a monofilament absorbable suture?

    a. Chromic gut

    b. Polypropylene

    c. Nylon

    d. Vicryl

106. Which of the following suture gauges is the smallest?

    a. 0

    b. 5-0

    c. 11-0

d. #2

107. Suture needles are categorized as three types: cutting, blunt, and tapered. How many variations of these types are there?
   a. 3
   b. 5
   c. 6
   d. 10

108. Which of the following spore is the most resistant?
   a. Viral
   b. Bacterial
   c. Fungal
   d. Tuberculosis

109. Which of the following best describes the difference between turnover OR suite cleaning and terminal OR suite cleaning?
   a. Turnover is done at the beginning and terminal at the end of the day
   b. Terminal is cleaning between each case, and turnover is done at the end of the day
   c. Terminal cleaning is the thorough cleaning done at the end of the day, while turnover is the cleaning done between cases
   d. These two terms mean the same thing and are interchangeable

110. What are the three types of sterilants?
   a. Thermal, chemical, radiation
   b. Thermal, physical, radiation
   c. Physical, chemical, steam
   d. Chemical, biological, steam

111. What are the two types of thermal sterilizing agents?
   a. Moist heat and dry heat
   b. Steam and cool air
   c. Dry and cold air
   d. Steam without pressure and hot air

112. Which of the following is a type of chemical sterilizing agent?
   a. Steam
   b. Ethylene oxide
   c. Microwave
   d. X ray

113. What is the difference between chemical and biological indicators?
   a. Chemical indicators indicate sterility for instruments, and biological indicators are for implants
   b. Both indicate sterility but for different agents, chemical for chemical and biological for radiation
   c. Chemical indicators do not ensure sterility and only show that the parameters of the sterilizer have been met, but biological indicators test for actual sterility through the use of resistant spores
   d. Chemical indicators ensure sterility of instruments, and biological indicators test for proper function of the autoclaves

114. Which of the following is the minimum frequency that biological indicators should be run in the sterilizers?
   a. Once a day
   b. Once a week and with all implants
   c. Once a month
   d. Bimonthly and with all implants

115. What does a positive (+) biological indicator mean?
   a. Sterility is guaranteed
   b. Sterility is not guaranteed
   c. All contained spores were killed
   d. The sterilizer cycle met all anticipated parameters

116. You are circulating a laparoscopic cholecystectomy, and the surgeon asks you for a Veress needle. What is the purpose of this device?
   a. To insert local anesthetic into the surgical field
   b. To insufflate the abdominal cavity
   c. To aspirate the gallbladder
   d. To insert the trocar into the abdominal cavity

117. Pfannenstiel incisions are mostly commonly used for which of the following surgeries?
   a. Appendectomy
   b. Exploratory laparotomy
   c. Abdominal hysterectomy
   d. Thoracotomy

118. The primary use for a McBurney incision is in which of the following surgeries?
   a. Appendectomy
   b. Exploratory laparotomy
   c. Vaginal hysterectomy
   d. Thoracotomy

119. Which of the following patients would be a candidate for bariatric surgery?
   a. A 40-year-old female with a BMI of 30 with mild comorbidities
   b. A 45-year-old male with a BMI of 45 and no other complications
   c. A 30-year-old female with a BMI of 35 with no other complications
   d. None of the above patients are candidates for this surgery

120. Which of the following would be a postoperative complication specific to below-the-knee amputations?
    a. Postoperative bleeding
    b. Phantom limb syndrome
    c. Flexion contracture
    d. Poor stump care

121. Endometrial ablation is a procedure using a heated probe for which one of the following procedures?
    a. Menorrhagia
    b. Breast cancer
    c. Peripheral vascular disease
    d. Bartholin cyst

122. Cardiac murmurs are graded on which of the following scales?
    a. I to IV
    b. A through D
    c. 1 to 6
    d. Acute to traumatic

123. While examining a patient preoperatively, you hear a cardiac murmur on systole. Which of the following will cause a systolic murmur?
    a. Aortic valve stenosis
    b. Aortic valve regurgitation
    c. Mitral valve stenosis
    d. Tricuspid valve stenosis

124. You are recovering a patient after an aortic valve replacement surgery. Which of the following is the most common cardiac arrhythmia after this type of surgery?
    a. Bradycardia
    b. Tachycardia
    c. Atrial fibrillation
    d. Heart block

125. You are performing your preoperative assessment on a 68-year-old male who is scheduled for an elective coronary artery bypass graft (CABG) surgery. Which of the following home medications should the patient not have stopped before surgery?
    a. Plavix
    b. Warfarin
    c. Lasix
    d. Aspirin

126. Cardiac output is made up of the patient's heart rate and which other factor?
    a. Pedal pulse
    b. Stroke volume
    c. Respiratory rate
    d. Glasgow coma scale

127. You are the circulating RN during a cardiac surgery. The anesthesia care provider tells you she will be performing a transesophageal echocardiography (TEE). What is the primary purpose of this procedure?
    a. To monitor wedge pressures
    b. To monitor myocardial ischemia
    c. To monitor myocardial infarction
    d. To evaluate esophageal tears

128. Beck's triad is made up of high jugular venous pressure, low arterial pressure, and quiet heart sounds. These symptoms are indicative of which syndrome?
    a. Increased intracranial pressure
    b. Pneumothorax
    c. Acute cardiac tamponade
    d. Cardiac asystole

129. Which of the following are potential complications of a mediastinoscopy?
    a. Recurrent laryngeal nerve injury
    b. Pulmonary edema
    c. Cardiac tamponade
    d. Esophageal tears

130. Which of the following complications is associated with thoracotomy but not video-assisted thoracoscopy (VAT)?
    a. Infection
    b. Spinal cord injury
    c. Bleeding
    d. Pneumothorax

131. Which of the following is an intravenous general anesthetic commonly given to children?
    a. Versed
    b. Demerol
    c. Ketamine
    d. Suprane

132. A thyroglossal duct cystectomy would be performed in which of the following positions?
    a. Supine
    b. Lithotomy
    c. Prone
    d. Lateral

133. Which of the following instrument trays would be most helpful during an indirect inguinal herniorrhaphy surgery?
    a. Abdominal hysterectomy tray
    b. Artery tray
    c. Minor instrument tray
    d. Minor rib tray

134. A pancreaticoduodenectomy is also known as what type of surgery?
   a. Whipple procedure
   b. Cholecystectomy
   c. Sigmoidoscopy
   d. Nissen procedure

135. For which condition would a laparoscopic Nissen fundoplication be most useful?
   a. Stomach cancer
   b. Hiatal hernia
   c. Femoral hernia
   d. Uterine fibroids

136. What is the purpose of a pyloroplasty?
   a. Increase peripheral blood flow to the lower extremities
   b. Increase gastric emptying
   c. Open the common bile duct
   d. Decrease gastric acid

137. What does the acronym ESWL stand for?
   a. External shock wave ligation
   b. Extracorporeal shock wave ligation
   c. Extracorporeal shock wave lithotripsy
   d. External shock wave lithotripsy

138. Your patient is scheduled for a decortication of the right lung. What does this mean?
   a. A lobe of the right lung is going to be removed
   b. Restrictive tissue is going to be stripped from this lung
   c. A chest tube is going to be placed to remove fluid from the right lung
   d. A wedge biopsy is going to be performed on this lung

139. A thymectomy is most commonly performed through which type of incision?
   a. Abdominal incision
   b. Sternal splitting incision
   c. Posterolateral chest incision
   d. Midline neck incision

140. In which of the following procedures would a Javid shunt be utilized?
   a. Thyroidectomy
   b. Aortic bifemoral bypass
   c. Carotid endarterectomy
   d. Cholecystectomy

141. When conducting a surgery using a laser, how should the laser be handled when not in use?
   a. Turn it off
   b. Place it on standby
   c. Be sure it is not facing any team members
   d. No special handling is required

142. Which of the following single-use items should not be reprocessed?
    a. Sutures
    b. Trocars
    c. Endoscopic graspers
    d. Opened and unused staplers

143. You are circulating a laparoscopic surgery, and you see the surgeon lay the light cord on the sterile drape. Which of the following would be the most effective action to prevent injury?
    a. Turn off the endoscopic tower
    b. Turn the light on standby
    c. Tell the surgeon to move the light off the sterile drape
    d. Nothing needs to be done in this situation

144. Before processing a bronchoscope in the peracetic acid sterilizing system, you should do which of the following?
    a. Make sure all the secretions are dried
    b. Perform a leak test
    c. Run powdered detergent through the channels and allow it to sit for 10 minutes
    d. Close all the channels so the fluid cannot get inside the scope

145. A Maryland dissector forcep would most commonly be used in which of the following surgeries?
    a. Lumbar laminectomy
    b. Vaginal hysterectomy
    c. Laparoscopic cholecystectomy
    d. Thyroidectomy

146. A cystotomy is an opening made into which organ?
    a. Bladder
    b. Heart
    c. Lung
    d. Uterus

147. A Marshall–Marchetti procedure is performed for what type of condition?
    a. Aortic valve stenosis
    b. Stress incontinence
    c. Cystocele
    d. Rectal fissure

148. In which of the following procedures might a Litvak Pereyra needle be used?
    a. Spinal anesthesia
    b. Abdominal aortic aneurysm repair
    c. Bladder neck suspension
    d. Epidural anesthesia

149. What is the purpose of a UNOS number?
    a. It is used for surgical billing
    b. It is used to identify appropriate bone implants assigned during a surgery
    c. It is the anonymous number given to trauma patients
    d. It is the identification number assigned to living and cadaver transplant organs

150. ViaSpan is used in which of the following procedures?
    a. Coronary artery bypass graft (CABG) surgery
    b. Heart catheterization
    c. Living-donor nephrectomy
    d. Pancreas transplant

151. When is a post-transplant patient at the most risk for infection?
    a. In the first three days after surgery
    b. The first two weeks after the transplant
    c. The first year after the transplant
    d. One to six months post-transplant

152. The Perioperative Patient Focused Model is divided into how many quadrants?
    a. Three
    b. Four
    c. Six
    d. Eight

153. In relation to surgical attire, which of the following is correct?
    a. It should be flammable
    b. It should always be disposable
    c. It should be low linting
    d. It can be reworn if not soiled

154. What is the primary purpose of wearing surgical attire?
    a. To distinguish to the patient you are the surgical RN
    b. To prevent bacterial shedding
    c. To act as personal protective equipment
    d. To prevent the spread of communicable diseases

155. You have removed a warm bottle of normal saline from your facility's fluid warmer. At the end of the surgery, you did not use the fluid. What should you do with it?
    a. Put it back in the warmer
    b. Change the expiration date to account for the time it was removed from the warmer
    c. Label the bottle "Do Not Rewarm," and store at room temperature
    d. Discard it

156. Which of the following is the appropriate way to warm irrigation fluids?
    a. Microwave
    b. Autoclave
    c. Warming cabinet or portable fluid warmer
    d. Warm blanket

157. You are the circulating RN preparing for a hysteroscopy. The surgeon has requested Dextran as the fluid media. Which of the following would be a potential contraindication to using this fluid?
    a. Monopolar electrosurgery
    b. Renal disease
    c. Allergy to shellfish
    d. Allergy to beet sugar

158. In which of the following surgeries would you possibly use 3% sorbitol as a fluid media?
a. Hysteroscopy
b. Laparoscopic cholecystectomy
c. Cystoscopy
d. Laparoscopic salpingo-oopherectomy

159. Which of the following is the most important reason to record the amount of fluid infused and the amount returned during a hysteroscopy?
a. So the patient does not get an infection
b. To prevent a distended bladder
c. Because fluids can be absorbed and cause severe complications
d. To correctly determine blood loss

160. You are the circulating RN and must assist the surgeon with placement of his sterile gown. Which of the following is true regarding what area the circulator may touch on the surgeon's gown?
a. The external waist tie
b. The wrist ties
c. The internal waist ties
d. None of the ties

161. After tying the surgeon's gown, which of the following parts is passed to the circulating nurse to finish the tying process?
a. The neck ties
b. There are no additional steps to the tying process.
c. The internal waist tie
d. The external waist tie tag

162. If the external waist tie does not have a tag attached to it, what can it be placed in to pass it to the circulator?
a. Wrapped around a knife handle
b. The paper packaging of the sterile gloves
c. The ungloved hand of the surgeon
d. The cuff of the gown

163. If you are using a gas-powered pneumatic tourniquet, which of the following is an appropriate gas to use?
a. Compressed air
b. Carbon dioxide
c. Nitrous oxide
d. Oxygen

164. Any healthcare facility that procures and/or stores human tissue for transfer to another facility must do which of the following?
a. Register with the Department of Human Services (DHS) as a tissue bank
b. Register with the Food & Drug Administration (FDA) as a tissue bank
c. Establish themselves as a nonprofit facility
d. Store the tissue in pathology

165. How often should the minimum temperature of the tissue storage freezer should be checked?

a. Daily
b. Once a shift
c. Weekly
d. Monthly

166. Which of the following is a true statement regarding sponge counts?
    a. Sponge counts only need to be done before and after the procedure
    b. Sponge counts should be done whenever any team member leaves the room
    c. As long as you perform a sponge count at wound closure, you do not need to count for each
       cavity closure
    d. Sponge counts should be done at any permanent relief of either the scrub or circulating nurse

167. Which of the following items should not be used in the surgical wound?
    a. Lap sponges
    b. Ray-Tec sponges
    c. Radiopaque towels
    d. Nonradiopaque towels

168. When should you perform an instrument count in addition to sponge and sharp counts?
    a. Only on abdominal cases
    b. Only on trauma cases
    c. Any time there is a risk of a retained instrument
    d. Instrument counts are never necessary

169. Surgical team members who are routinely exposed to procedures using x rays, such as
orthopedic cases, and are less than two feet away from the radiation beam should wear which of
the following additional protective items?
    a. Thyroid shield
    b. Eye protection
    c. Laser mask
    d. Wrap-around lead aprons

170. You are the circulating nurse in an orthopedic procedure utilizing a C-arm device. The surgeon
asks for this device to be moved to another area of the patient's body. Which of the following
personnel may move this device?
    a. Only the circulating RN
    b. Any MD
    c. The orthopedic vendor
    d. The radiology tech

171. Surgical specimens are listed according to three categories for handling. Which of the following
best describes these categories?
    a. Surgical pathology, gross, disposal
    b. Frozen, permanent, gross
    c. Frozen, permanent, disposal
    d. Banking, surgical pathology, disposal

172. Forensic specimens, such as bullets, should be carefully handled and properly documented to
preserve which of the following?
    a. Chain of evidence

b. Chain of command
c. Chain of communication
d. Chain of custody

173. The scrub nurse pulls up which part of the gown when assisting the surgeon in gloving?
    a. The shoulder of the gown
    b. The waist of the gown
    c. The sleeves of the gown
    d. The neck of the gown

174. What is bariatric surgery performed for?
    a. Cancer
    b. Weight loss
    c. Fractures
    d. Renal failure

175. You are the circulating RN for a patient having a ventral hernia repair. During your preoperative assessment, you notice this patient is morbidly obese. Which one of the following is an associated disease with this condition?
    a. Type 1 diabetes
    b. Osteoporosis
    c. GERD
    d. Hypotension

176. Which of the following bariatric surgeries is a combination of the restrictive and malabsorption methods?
    a. Gastric banding
    b. Proximal gastric bypass
    c. Roux-en-Y gastric bypass
    d. Jejunoileal bypass

177. You are interviewing a patient preoperatively who is having an exploratory laparotomy for abdominal pain. In her surgical history, you note she had an adjustable gastric band placed three years ago. Which of the following is a complication specific to these procedures that might be contributing to her condition?
    a. Incisional hernia formation
    b. Anastomosis leakage
    c. Tissue erosion
    d. Anastomotic stricture

178. Knowing the required intraoperative positioning required for a gastric band placement, which of the following additional pieces of equipment would be necessary?
    a. Allen stirrups
    b. Footboard
    c. Shoulder roll
    d. Axillary roll

179. Laryngeal nerve paralysis is a potential complication of which block?
    a. Celiac block
    b. Intercostal block

c. Intraocular block

d. Brachial plexus

180. A scleral buckling surgery is performed for which disease condition?
   a. Retinal detachment
   b. Glaucoma
   c. Corneal lacerations
   d. Fuchs dystrophy

181. Labyrinthectomy is an otologic surgery performed for which condition?
   a. Hearing loss
   b. Severe vertigo
   c. Chronic ear infections
   d. Cholesteatoma

182. An Alvarado foot holder is used for which of the following procedures?
   a. Total hip arthroplasty
   b. Total knee arthroplasty
   c. Knee arthroscopy
   d. Femoral-popliteal bypass

183. What is a dermatome device used for?
   a. Removing valves from a vein graft
   b. Promoting bone growth in nonhealing fractures
   c. Removing tissue to be used in split-thickness skin grafts
   d. Locating sentinel lymph nodes

184. You are circulating a carotid endarectomy, and the surgeon asks for loupes. What is she asking for?
   a. Vessel loops
   b. Her magnifying eyeglasses
   c. Silk ties
   d. Hemaclips

185. As the circulating RN, you know that using proper draping materials is essential for patient protection. Which of the following best describes the current recommendations for choosing the correct draping material?
   a. The drapes must be resistant to fluid, tearing, puncture, and lint free to reduce contamination of the sterile field
   b. Different institutions decide on the guidelines that best suit their organizational needs and policies
   c. The current recommendations are under review, and they will be available in the upcoming year
   d. The drapes must be able to maintain the heat of the human body to avoid hypothermia during the surgical procedure

186. Which of the following describes a special consideration for correct draping that the scrub and circulating RN should be aware of?
   a. They should ensure that the prep solutions have dried before applying surgical drapes
   b. The scrubbed team members should hold the drapes below waist level

c. The surgeon should perform the procedure quickly to minimize potential infections

d. The scrubbed team members never cuff the drapes over gloved hands

187. When you are the scrub RN, and you are helping place the surgical drapes, you should be aware that once the drapes have been placed they should not be moved or readjusted. Which of the following best describes the rationale for this placement?

a. Shifting of a drape can potentially cause contamination

b. It reduces the cost of needing additional drapes

c. Repositioning a drape is an acceptable practice

d. Shifting of a drape can cause skin irritation

188. You are helping drape a patient for an appendectomy. You first drape the area planned for the incision, and then you work outward. Why are surgical drapes laid in this manner?

a. To visually maintain the correct anatomical positioning of the patient

b. To provide additional warmth during the surgical procedure

c. To reduce contamination

d. To verify that the correct site is being draped

189. In order to prevent injury to fellow team members, the scrub RN should pass loaded knife blades in which of the following manners?

a. With the blade toward the physician

b. With the blade off the handle

c. With a "hands-free" technique

d. With the blade in his/her hand

190. In order to lower the risk of surgical site infections, the doors to the OR suite should remain in which of the following positions?

a. Open if a surgery is in process

b. Closed as much as possible

c. Open if there is no surgery occurring

d. The position of the OR doors does not affect infection control

191. At the conclusion of a stable carotid endarectomy surgery, after extubation the anesthesia care provider may ask you, as the circulating RN, to get a laryngoscope or glidescope. Which of the following provides the best rationale for this request?

a. To emergently reintubate the patient

b. To check if the vocal cords are responding

c. To check for bleeding

d. To properly suction the patient

192. Immediately before beginning any procedure, what should the circulating nurse do?

a. Call a "time out" with all team members involved with the procedure

b. Identity the patient

c. Find sitting stools

d. Start an IV line

193. You are circulating a thoracic surgery, and the anesthesia care provider plans to perform an intercostal block. Which of the following is a potential complication of an intercostal nerve block?

a. Air embolism

b. Numbness

c. Headache

d. Horner syndrome

194. You are the preoperative RN, and you are conducting the anesthesia consent for a patient who will be getting a peripheral nerve block. Which of the following is a potential site for a peripheral nerve block?

a. Cerebrospinal fluid (CSF)

b. Epidural space

c. Digits

d. Earlobe

195. The circulating RN should be aware that an intravascular injection of local anesthesia from a peripheral nerve block can lead to which of the following?

a. Overdose and possible cardiac arrest

b. Numbness

c. Loss of the limb

d. Paralysis of the limb

196. You are the preoperative RN performing your assessment. You know the first thing you should do is properly identify the patient using two pieces of information specific to that person. Which of the following would be appropriate information that could be used for this purpose?

a. Name and date of birth

b. Name and weight

c. Name and age

d. Date of birth and favorite color

197. Which of the following complications are specific to arteriovenous (AV) fistula patients postoperatively?

a. Paralysis

b. Renal failure

c. Stroke

d. Hemorrhage at the surgical site

198. Which of the following documents should be reviewed in the preprocedure assessment to verify the procedure?

a. Patient's surgical consent form

b. Patient's insurance information

c. Advance directive

d. Medication record

199. After the circulating nurse reads the information for the "time out," all team members should do which of the following?

a. Verbalize agreement if it is correct

b. Ignore her

c. Start the procedure

d. Leave the room

200. Which of the following is an example of a neurovascular assessment that may be performed in the preoperative setting prior to the surgical procedure?

a. Nausea level

b. Pain level
c. Skin breakdown
d. Peripheral pulses

Answers and Explanations

1. B: Answers A and D are elements of the AORN Perioperative Patient Focused Model. Answer C is a human response pattern discussed by North American Nursing Diagnosis Association (NANDA). Planning is the only answer that is a step in the nursing process. Planning is needed to create the necessary interventions for the surgical patient, her problem, and potential problems. It is during this phase that caregivers should include the patient's input in their plan of care.

2. C: Although answer B should be discussed with the patient during the informed consent procedure, it is not the primary purpose. Informed consent does have a legal component and should be protected information, but its primary purpose is to inform the patient what is planned, the expected outcomes, and what are the alternatives. With the exception of emergencies, performing a procedure on a patient who has not been given proper informed consent can have legal consequences. All planned procedures should be listed on the consent form and should be addressed before the patient signs.

3. A: Although the preoperative and circulating RNs validate the consent form for correctness, it is the surgeon's responsibility to obtain informed consent. This is achieved by completely explaining the procedure to the patient in a manner she can understand, listing the risks, benefits, complications, and alternatives available. This conversation should also include what to expect postoperatively and which of the patient's lifestyle factors might affect the plan of care.

4. B: The patient return electrode "grounds" the patient from injury from the ESU current. Poor contact can prevent this function and even allow fluid to pool underneath it, leading to a possible burn. The tip of the ESU pencil can remain very hot between uses. Laying this tip on a surgical drape may start a fire. The ESU pencil should always be returned to its holder between uses. The patient return electrode should not be placed over a previous surgical site, if possible, because the electrical current could conduct through any metal implant that might exist at the site, or the tissue may already be compromised from poor wound healing. Finally, evidence-based practice shows alcohol-based preps to be very effective in the prevention of surgical site infections. It is safe to use this type of prep in the operating room as long as the manufacturer's recommendations are followed and the prep is dried completely before the surgical drape is applied.

5. C: Sutures, along with clips, clamps, and tourniquets are examples of manual hemostasis. The laser and ESU are thermal agents. Fibrin glue is a chemical hemostasis agent.

6. D: Type 1 diabetic patients have a potential for dehydration, electrolyte imbalance, and inadequate circulation. These factors, among others, can cause hypertension in these patients intraoperatively. Infection and delayed wound healing are potential postoperative complications with diabetic patients.

7. A: Congenital anomalies, trauma, and acquired disease processes are the most common indicators for surgery in children. Although answers b through d may cause the mortality of a pediatric patient, alone they do not act as indicators for surgery.

8. B: This age group tends to experience separation anxiety when separated from parents. Body image concerns are more appropriate in the teen years. Four to six year olds may act like fantasy

characters when confronted with stressful situations, and nonverbal sounds would be more appropriate for infant-age patients.

9. C: Answer A refers to the supine position, with the patient flat. Answer B describes the Trendelenburg position, and answer D is lithotomy positioning. Keeping the patient supine and elevating the entire head of the bed so it is higher than the foot is described as reverse Trendelenburg. This position would be requested in this particular surgery to provide better observation of the stomach and diaphragm.

10. C: Without proper padding and extremity placement, the lateral position can cause nerve damage to the extremities, such as the brachial plexus. Lower back strain could occur with lithotomy. Pressure ulcers to the back of the head would be more consistent with a supine position or some version of it. Skin tears on the buttocks result from shearing forces. These types of injuries are a risk of the reverse Trendelenburg position.

11. A: MS is not well absorbed by mouth (PO) and is not recommended. Answers C and D would be too large of a dose for a pediatric patient, although the appropriate dose could be given IV, IM, or SQ.

12. C: Nausea, vomiting, and respiratory depression are not considered therapeutic effects but rather side effects, which are not specific to midazolam hydrochloride (Versed) alone, but can occur with many medications. Although pain control can occur with the use of Versed, short-term amnesia of the pre- and intraoperative time is the medication's primary purpose for administration. Both the circulating and postanesthesia care nurse should be aware of this effect because it could be confusing for the patient, as he or she will often not even remember going into the operating suite.

13. B: Stenosis of the pulmonary valve, not aortic valve, is one of the four defects found in tetralogy of Fallot. Babies experience poor oxygen circulation due to these defects and are often referred to as "blue babies." Hypertrophy to the right ventricle and displacement of the aorta to the right are the corrections to answers c and d.

14. D: Elderly patients may have more drug interactions because their tolerance and detoxification through the kidneys and liver are often lower than in their younger counterparts. Because this population often has lower body fat as well, fat-soluble medications, such as many anesthetic agents, may metabolize slower and cause a dangerous interaction with pain control medications.

15. D: The operating room department is made up of three areas: unrestricted, semirestricted, and restricted. In the unrestricted areas, such as the front office, you can wear street clothes. In semirestricted areas, which usually refer to areas inside the department but not inside the suite, you need to wear authorized scrub attire and hair covering. A mask is not required in these areas. The restricted areas include anywhere that sterile supplies are opened, such as the actual OR suite. In these areas, proper attire and a mask must be worn.

16. A: Although the temperature may be adjusted for patient safety, 68°–73° F is the recommended temperature range to keep the patient normothermic. Warmer temperatures may increase the growth of harmful organisms in the surgical suite. In addition, humidity may be affected by temperature changes outside this optimal range. Increases in humidity can also harbor microorganism growth.

17. C: The optimal score with the Aldrete postanesthesia scoring system is a 10. There are five areas that are assessed; each is scored 0–2 points. Although this patient is fully awake, moving, and back to preanesthetic circulatory function, she is not breathing deeply and still needs oxygen to keep her saturation above 92. These last two areas would be scored as a 1 instead of the optimal 2, giving the patient an Aldrete score of 8.

18. C: Only areas from the chest to the sterile field, and two inches above the elbow and gloves are sterile. The back of the gown and below the waist are not considered sterile.

19. B: Only the top of a sterilely draped back table is actually considered sterile, not the edges or sides. Any sterile item that extends past the edge of the sterile area is no longer considered sterile and should be discarded immediately. Although the sterile scrub tech would not want to touch the contaminated tip, she can discard it by touching the part still on the table or remove it from the field so the circulator can discard it. A nonsterile person should never reach over or onto a sterile field to retrieve an item.

20. D: The minimum recommended distance is 12 inches or 1 foot. Although answer A is a correct option, it is not the minimum distance asked for in the question. This distance is the agreed-upon "safe" distance by perioperative professional organizations so as to prevent inadvertent contamination.

21. B: This is the recommended method by perioperative professional organizations to open sterile items. Loose edges could fold back and contaminate the instrument or field because the inside wrapper is only considered sterile up to 1 inch from the edge. As a result, the person opening should keep control of the flaps in her hand as she opens. In this question, the scrub tech is already sterile, so she cannot open the instrument because the outside of the wrap is not sterile.

22. B: You should open the door and leave the items inside to dry. Fifteen to sixty minutes is the recommended drying time for steam sterilizers, but this range varies by manufacturer. You would not want to remove the items and put them away or leave them on a table because the items will still be very warm. Placing them on a cold surface could cause condensation on the surface and put the items at risk for contamination from strike-through of the collected fluid. There is no separate "dry" cycle for these sterilizers.

23. A: Although it could happen to any of these instruments, you shouldn't place a needle holder on an instrument magnet because it could become magnetized. Because the purpose of this instrument is to safely manipulate suture needles, if the instrument becomes magnetized it may not properly release the needle or attract it back and cause injury to the sterile team or the patient.

24. A: Of the four choices, only an ESU uses electrical current to manipulate the patient's tissues. In order to complete the electrical circuit and not harm the patient, electricity flows from the unit (generator) to the active electrode (Bovie pencil) and is returned to the generator by the return patient electrode, also known as the inactive dispersive electrode, rather than through the patient or team members.

25. B: Allogenous refers to blood that is collected from a donor other than oneself. Blood substitutes are oxygen-carrying products that are alternatives to giving actual blood, whereas blood volume expanders only add volume and have no oxygen-carrying component. Autologous blood transfusions, or autotransfusion, refers to collecting a patient's own blood and returning it to them.

This can be achieved through a preoperative donation or intraoperatively with the use of a blood salvage unit.

26. B: Although all are personal safety equipment, eyewear should be specific for the laser used because the eye can absorb the laser beams. The use of a tight-fitting laser mask, not an N-95 mask, would be appropriate.

27. A: Warning signs should be placed so anyone entering the room will know that the laser is in use. Although you should not store liquids on the laser equipment, the scrub tech should have a bowl of sterile water or saline solution available in case of a fire. When the laser is not in use, it should be kept in "standby," even if the surgeon requests it to remain armed. This is to prevent inadvertent firing that could injure the patient or team. Finally, a halon extinguisher, not an ABC-type extinguisher should be available.

28. A: NPO stands for nil per os, or nothing by mouth. This is important in the perioperative setting because food or liquids ingested less than eight hours prior to surgery can be regurgitated and aspirated under anesthesia.

29. D: All of the above items should be removed before surgery, but only the nail polish/acrylic nail choice can interfere with the anesthesia monitoring of the patient. Many pulse oximeters, used for oxygen saturation monitoring, are placed on the finger and require visualization of the nail bed to properly function. Nail bed color is also used as an indicator of peripheral circulation. The patient should be instructed that if she wears these items, she should uncover at least one fingernail.

30. C: All of these items should be addressed in your preoperative assessment, but first you should make sure you have the right patient. You cannot just do this by asking the patient's name because there are often patients with the same or similar names. Hence, a demographic piece of information, such as date of birth, should also be verified. This information should be compared with the patient's armband, and the correct spelling is verified. If the patient cannot verbally answer, then staff or visitors accompanying the patient to the preoperative area should do this verification.

31. C: Many herbal medications can cause interactions with intraoperative medications and should be noted. Ginkgo biloba can increase bleeding, not cardiac arrhythmias. It is usually not substantial enough to delay or cancel surgery, but the physicians caring for the patient should be made aware that she is taking ginkgo biloba, so they may plan accordingly.

32. D: The ASA physical status classification system has six classes. Healthy patients are ASA I. ASA II is mild disease, III is severe, IV is life threatening, and V applies to patients that are not expected to live more than 24 hours. Answer C would be ASA VI.

33. C: Although urine may be needed to perform lab work prior to surgery, the main reason patients without a Foley catheter already in place are encouraged to void is to prevent bladder distention and incontinence, because an anesthetized patient cannot feel the urge to urinate. This is very important in abdominal surgeries, because an enlarged bladder could be damaged during surgery. The pooled fluid from an incontinent patient could also cause skin damage.

34. C: Shellfish allergy can indicate an allergy to iodine. Many contrast media contain iodine. Contrast is a necessary component in endovascular procedures due to the use of x ray. This would not affect antibiotic choice or be indicative of a latex allergy. An allergy to eggs might affect the use of propofol.

35. C: The missing component is right time.

36. A: Versed is a benzodiazepine. Romazicon, also known as Flumazenil, is the only benzodiazepine antagonist in this group. Narcan, also known as Naloxone hydrochloride, would be appropriate for narcotic reversal. Although Benadryl might be helpful for an allergic reaction, it will not reverse the effects of a benzodiazepine. Epinephrine would be helpful in an arrest situation as well, but it will not reverse the effects either.

37. C: Intraoperative awareness is the rare condition in which a patient seems to be under anesthesia, but she can still hear and feel what is happening during surgery. This is affected by the depth of anesthesia, a difficult thing to monitor at times. There are now monitoring techniques such as bispectral index (BIS) monitoring that can sense the patient's brain waves through an electrode placed on the forehead. Based on the number reading, the anesthesia care provider can better determine the patient's level of consciousness.

38. A: The BIS monitor has a range in readings from 100 to 0. A 100 reading on the BIS monitor means the patient is fully awake, and 0 is no brain activity.

39. C: Nerve, epidural, and intrathecal blocks are all forms of regional anesthesia.

40. C: Bupivacaine, or Marcaine, is a common local anesthetic medication used in epidural anesthesia. Meperidine is a narcotic. Bacitracin is an antibiotic, and succinylcholine is a paralytic agent used as a muscle relaxant in general anesthesia.

41. C: A double-cuff tourniquet is used for this procedure. In a Bier block, once the tourniquet is placed, the patient's arm is elevated and wrapped with a compression bandage (Esmarch) to remove blood from the distal portion of the extremity. The upper cuff of the tourniquet is then inflated. The local medication is injected through an intravenous line in that extremity. Once the medication has anesthetized the extremity, the lower cuff of the tourniquet is inflated, and the upper cuff is released.

42. D: You would want to slowly release the tourniquet so the body can absorb any remaining local anesthesia. A bolus of this medication could lead to cardiac or central nervous system toxicity. There should not be excessive bleeding or pain with this type of anesthesia.

43. D: You should always start counting items on the surgical field, and then the back table, followed by the items that have been passed off the surgical field, also referred to as the floor count. Counting in a consistent manner, starting at the surgical field will help prevent delays in wound closure and miscounts.

44. A: The medications given to the patient for general anesthesia can be very disorienting and frightening for the patient. It is important for the circulating nurse to stay at the bedside to comfort the patient and to assist the anesthesia provider as needed in case there is a complication.

45. C: Cricoid pressure helps block the esophagus to prevent aspiration of gastric contents. This would be especially important for a patient with a history of gastroesophageal reflux disease (GERD), because he would be at additional risk of aspiration. Cricoid has no purpose in keeping the neck stable. Closing off the esophagus actually helps the anesthesia care provider better visualize the vocal cords, a necessary landmark when intubating a patient with an endotracheal (ET) tube.

46. C: Although the other answers may be true, in relation to the intubation process, C is the best answer. Moving the patient before the anesthesia provider has approved may lead to accidental extubation and loss of the patient's airway, which can be life threatening.

47. C: Sudden revascularization of the operative limb in fem-pop bypass patients may lead to operative leg swelling. Although the other answers are possible complications, they are very rare.

48. B: Because of the need of thoracic cross clamping during these surgeries, the spinal cord may become ischemic from the lack of blood flow. This is especially true if the cross clamping lasts longer than 30 minutes. The patient's risk of stroke or previous spine surgery would be an additional patient-specific risk factor, not on associated with the procedure itself.

49. C: Frequent monitoring of vital signs will help the PACU nurse identify any complications in a timely manner. Each hospital may have a policy regarding vital sign monitoring, such as every 5 minutes for the first 20 minutes, then every 15 minutes throughout the postoperative stay. Others may require vitals every 5 minutes throughout the entire first hour. In relation to the other answers, every 5 minutes would be the most appropriate for a new postoperative patient.

50. A: Although all of these answers are recorded for a surgical patient, only the dermatome levels are specific to regional anesthetic patients. This is to determine the level of the anesthetic as it wears off postoperatively.

51. A: Shivering increases cardiac demand and may lead to cardiac ischemia and arrest in this vascular surgery patient, especially due to her already-compromised cardiac status.

52. B: Although blankets and warm IV fluids are helpful in warming a patient, the use of forced-air warming blankets have been shown to be the most effective in warming hypothermic patients. These devices have been found to be useful in pre-, intra-, and postoperative areas.

53. C: Any vascular surgery that requires catheter placement, such as a pacemaker, may need a chest x ray postoperatively to verify proper placement. This is usually done in the PACU area. Although this patient might require additional lines or a blood transfusion due to her overall disease process, it would not be a routine order for a pacemaker placement patient.

54. B: To prevent the risk of needle sticks, sharps are always placed in a puncture-proof container specifically designed for them, not any type of trash bag. Because the sharps discussed in this question cannot be reprocessed, you would not put them in a container to be resterilized.

55. C: According to current National Patient Safety Goals and the Surgical Care Improvement Project (SCIP), antibiotics should be administered within 1 hour of incision for best practice effectiveness.

56. A: Limiting the number of persons going in and out of the OR suite helps to lower the number of microbes allowed to enter the room. This, paired with proper air exchanges and other environmental controls, helps reduce surgical-site infections.

57. A: Supination, or palms facing up, when the arms are extended helps to prevent ulnar nerve damage in the supine position. All other answers could result in injury.

58. C: A wedge under the patient's right side helps relieve uterine pressure off the vena cava.

59. B: It is important to document everyone present in the positioning of the patient because the patient's chart is a legal document. This information could become important should the patient sustain an injury attributed to the positioning during the surgery.

60. D: Gel has been found to be more helpful in the prevention of pressure sore formation than the traditional foam mattress. Gel is supportive to pressure points, where foam collapses. These mattresses are also less likely to crack like their foam counterparts, which can cause skin damage and create potential for infection.

61. A: Smoking causes vasoconstriction and thereby compromises blood flow to the periphery of the body and puts the tissues at risk. This places these patients at a higher risk for ulcer formation.

62. C: Risk increases the longer the surgery is, but studies show it dramatically increases after three hours. If possible, efforts should be made to reposition the patient after this time. If this is not possible, careful inspection and documentation of the skin integrity should take place when the surgery ends.

63. B: You should use the wrapper of the sterile gown to create a sterile surface away from the patient and the sterile back table. This is to prevent contamination of the sterile field by falling droplets from your wet hands or inadvertently touching sterile items when picking up your gown and gloves.

64. B: If you will be gowning and gloving yourself, you should not open your supplies on the back table, in order to prevent contamination. It is acceptable to open these supplies on the back table if someone else, who is already wearing sterile supplies, will assist you so you are not required to touch the sterile back table to retrieve your supplies.

65. A: Supplies without a posted expiration date are considered sterile until the package is opened or integrity is compromised. This is called "event-related" sterility.

66. A: Holding the drapes above the OR table prevents the edges from being contaminated. Draping should start from the site and proceed outward, because the site is sterile and the other areas are not.

67. A: Nonsterile equipment is sometimes needed for a procedure. If it can be sterilized, then you should do so. If not, the best option is to cover it with a sterile drape to prevent contamination to the sterile field. Many vendors make drapes for specific items used in surgery that cannot be sterilized, such as C-arm drapes.

68. D: Once an item has expired, there is no way to guarantee its sterility, and it should not be used on the sterile field to prevent contamination and surgical-site infection. Even if it is an emergency situation, a substitute item should be used.

69. B: The edges of solution containers are considered contaminated once the solutions have been poured, so they cannot be recapped for reuse, even if the cap was kept sterile.

70. A: The safety strap helps secure the patient, preventing falls, and it should be placed across her thighs. A strap across the chest could impede respirations and is not as secure. Due to the narrow width of most OR tables, a safety strap should be placed whether the patient is sedated or not, even

- 87 -

if other staff is available to secure her. Should the patient move unexpectedly, she could still fall and injury herself and the staff members who try to catch her.

71. B: If a patient can physically assist with transfer, a minimum of two staff members are needed to stand on either side of the bed to prevent falls. If the patient is unable to assist, then a minimum of four team members are needed.

72. B: After 30 minutes, blood products requiring refrigeration can no longer be returned to the blood bank, because the cells have already started to break down.

73. C: If you suspect a blood reaction, you should immediately stop the transfusion. You should then return any unused blood to the blood bank for investigation.

74. C: Any two licensed professionals may check the blood products before administration. This can be the circulating RN and the anesthesia care provider or two RNs. It does not need to be your patient to assist in verifying blood products.

75. C: The circulating nurse should report all deaths in the OR to the coroner's office for review. This information can usually be found on the "death packet" paperwork or in the facility's policy for management of death in the operating room. No lines or drains should be removed from the patient until the coroner's office has released the patient. This is especially important for cases where criminal activity may have been involved.

76. B: Postmortem identification tags are specific to identification of deceased patients. One should be placed on the patient, usually on the toe, and another on the outside of the shroud.

77. B: The scrub nurse carefully picks up the towel by a corner, with one hand. This is to prevent water from dropping on the towel and contaminating it.

78. A: The scrub nurse should dry from the fingers upward without retracing an area. This helps to prevent contamination of the cleansed areas.

79. D: Per JCAHO recommendations, the person with the most knowledge of the patient and planned procedure should mark the patient. This is usually the surgeon.

80. A: A permanent skin marker should be used so the marking is not removed during the skin prep.

81. D: In order to avoid confusion, it is recommended that the surgeon write his initials on the surgical site. Other methods can be confusing and lead to a wrong-site surgery.

82. B: Although this information should be verified with the patient in the preoperative area, the final "time out" should be immediately before the procedure starts, after draping, and it should be repeated for each additional procedure. It is important to be sure that any surgical site marks are visible after draping so they may be verified in the time-out process.

83. A: When a patient is placed prone, or on her stomach, chest rolls are used to help relieve the weight on the chest. This allows for better lung expansion and adequate breathing. Stirrups are used for lithotomy positions. Footboards are useful in reverse Trendelenburg positioning, and beanbags are mostly used in lateral positions.

84. C: Jackknife positioning is another name for the Kraske position.

85. C: In the Kraske position, the patient is placed prone and the foot of the bed is lowered. Then the entire bed is tilted so the patient's hips are higher than the rest of the body. This position greatly increases visualization in rectal surgery cases. Answer A would be in the lithotomy position. Answers B and D would be supine.

86. C: Surgical skin preps are meant to reduce the skin flora as much as possible by cleaning and chemically decontaminating the tissue. There is no way to sterilize or completely eliminate the skin flora. There are specific products that are used to degrease the skin, when necessary. Some surgical prep products have a degreaser product in them, but that is not the primary purpose of the prep.

87. D: Of the parts listed, the umbilicus is considered a contaminated area. If it will be included in the surgical field, such as an abdominal surgery, it should be prepped first; otherwise, contaminates could be dragged out and disrupt the already-prepped site. In this case, surgical swabs soaked in appropriate surgical prep are usually used to clean the umbilicus, and then the rest of the abdomen is prepped.

88. C: Because the recipient site is considered contaminated in this case; it should be prepped last to prevent inadvertent contamination of the donor site. It is recommended to use a colorless prep, so the surgeon can evaluate the vascular supply to the donor skin. If there is not proper vascularity, the donor skin will not survive on the recipient site.

89. A: Chlorhexidine gluconate is the only antiseptic solution on this list that is an ingredient in many surgical preps. Acetone is used as an effective degreaser, but by itself it does not have antiseptic qualities. ChloraPrep is actually a skin prep product that is made up of chlorhexidine gluconate and alcohol.

90. C: This test takes a muscle biopsy and exposes it to caffeine and halothane to check for an MH-like reaction. This test should be performed preoperatively if the patient is at risk for an MH event.

91. A: Dantrolene use has reduced the mortality associated with an MH crisis from 70% to less than 10%.

92. B: Symptoms of MH can reoccur for up to 72 hours after an incident.

93. D: You give 2.5 mg/kg IV initially and repeat dosing until signs and symptoms abate. You may need to increase the concentration to stop the signs and symptoms from continuing.

94. D: Hyperkalemia is a serious side effect of MH. It can cause serious cardiac dysrhythmias and renal damage. Using fluids containing potassium will increase the already-elevated serum potassium levels, causing further serious side effects.

95. D: Oral intake is not given in the Phase I area, so the return of the gag reflex is not normally tested in this area, but it is in Phase II. From this area, patients are usually discharged home or to some other off-site care facility, and it is essential that the patient can tolerate fluids, if she did preoperatively.

96. D: Because the effects of any regional anesthesia should be worn off by the time the patient reaches Phase II, motor and sensory function are not a normal assessment area.

97. A: A fenestrated drape is the formal name for a drape with openings. These openings can be in a variety of shapes and in multiple locations.

98. B: Carbon dioxide is used to insufflate the abdomen during laparoscopic cases. The other gases listed would be toxic to the patient if used in this manner.

99. B: The insufflated CO2 gas is measured in mm Hg, and although the intra-abdominal pressure may be adjusted by the surgeon to better meet the needs of the patient, the recommended level is 12–15mm Hg.

100. A: The CO2 gas insufflated into the abdomen causes a space to be formed in the cavity, so the surgeon can better visualize the internal structures and have space to work.

101. A: The surgeon and/or the anesthesia care provider are the healthcare professionals who should determine the appropriate setting of pressure when using a pneumatic tourniquet due to the potential harm to the patient.

102. C: The pressure setting for upper extremities is usually 30–70mmHg above the patient's systolic pressure. This has been found to be acceptable to control blood loss but limit damage to the occluded tissues.

103. D: In order to reduce damage to the limb, after each hour of surgery the limb should be evaluated. The tourniquet may be deflated briefly to restore blood flow to the limb as needed during these one-hour evaluations. This is especially important during very lengthy surgeries, because the tissue will die without proper blood circulation.

104. D: Vicryl is the only multifilament suture listed. Multifilament sutures should not be used in infected sites because they have a characteristic referred to as capillarity, which can cause the suture to harbor bacteria and fluids.

105. A: Chromic gut is the only one from the list that is both a monofilament and an absorbable suture. Nylon and polypropylene (Prolene) are nonabsorbable. Vicryl, although absorbable, is a multifilament suture.

106. C: Suture is sized according to gauge, similar to sewing thread. The largest gauge is #5, and the smallest is 11-0. The most commonly used sizes are #1- 4-0.

107. B: There are five variations of these three categories: conventional cutting, reverse cutting, side cutting, tapered, and blunt.

108. B: Bacterial spores are the most resistant due to their capacity to withstand external destructive agents.

109. C: The main differences between these two types of OR suite cleaning is that turnover cleaning is done between each surgery, and terminal cleaning is done at the end of the day and is a more complete cleaning.

110. A: Thermal, chemical, and radiation are the three types of sterilants. Physical is not a type. Steam is a form of thermal.

111. A: Moist heat (steam under pressure) and dry heat are the two types of thermal agents. Cool or cold air are not thermal options.

112. B: Ethylene oxide, EO, is the only type of chemical agent listed. Steam is a form of thermal agent. Microwave and X ray are forms of radiation agents.

113. C: Chemical indicators test the conditions within the sterilizer. These indicators do not indicate sterility, just that the parameters of the sterilization cycle have been met. Biological indicators are the only way to assure sterility, because they have living spores inside that are resistant to sterilizing agents. The biological indicators are tested after the cycle, and if the contained spores are dead, it proves that the item is truly sterile.

114. B: To ensure that the sterilizers are properly sterilizing products, biological indicators should be run in them at least once a week. Implants should always have a bio run with them to ensure sterility before they are placed in a patient.

115. B: If the biological indicator is read positive, that means all the contained spores were not killed and sterility is not guaranteed.

116. B: CO_2 gas is inserted into an abdominal cavity either through a percutaneous method using a Veress needle or by the open technique using a trocar.

117. C: A Pfannenstiel incision is a lower abdominal incision usually just above or within the pubic hairline. It is a good incision for pelvic surgeries and is used primarily for cesarean sections and abdominal hysterectomies.

118. A: A McBurney incision is an abdominal incision in the right lower quadrant. Although it is a quick incision, it is muscle splitting; therefore, it is primarily used for appendectomy cases where its limited exposure is appropriate.

119. B: A person with a body mass index of 40 or above, or 35 to 40 with serious comorbidities would be a potential candidate for bariatric surgery.

120. C: All the answers could be possible complications of all amputations, but flexion contractures are specific to below-the-knee amputations. As a result, many surgeons may choose to splint the operative leg postoperatively and order special exercises to prevent this.

121. A: During endometrial ablation, a heated probe is inserted into the uterine cavity to treat menorrhagia, or dysfunctional bleeding.

122. C: These murmurs are graded on a scale of 1 to 6. These grades are determined by the murmur's loudness from very faint to audible without the stethoscope completely touching the chest.

123. A: Aortic valve stenosis will cause a murmur on systole, whereas the other choices would present as diastole murmurs.

124. D: Heart blocks are the most common arrhythmia after aortic valve surgery. Bradycardia can indicate right coronary artery occlusion. Atrial fibrillation may indicate mitral valve disease.

125. D: Plavix is usually stopped within 48 hours of cardiac surgery. Warfarin, also known as Coumadin, should be stopped 5 to 7 days prior to surgery. Diuretics, such as Lasix, should be stopped the morning of surgery, but it is usually not necessary to stop aspirin prior to this surgery.

126. B: Cardiac output (CO) is determined by the heart rate (HR) times the stroke volume (SV). Stroke volume is the amount of blood returned from the heart after each contraction. The equation commonly used to represent this is $CO = HR \times SV$.

127. B: TEE monitoring is an invasive tool that is the best way to monitor myocardial ischemia. It can also be useful in cardiac valve surgeries, examining the problems before and the effectiveness of the repair after.

128. C: Beck's triad is an indicator of an acute cardiac tamponade.

129. A: Infection, hemorrhage, pneumothorax, and recurrent laryngeal nerve injury are all possible complications of mediastinoscopic surgery.

130. B: Spinal cord injury is the only listed complication that is not also shared by VAT surgery.

131. C: Ketamine is the only answer that is both given intravenously and is a general anesthetic agent.

132. A: A thyroglossal duct cystectomy is the excision of a duct and cyst inferior to the hyoid bone in the middle of the neck. Positioning for this type of surgery is similar to a thyroidectomy. The patient is supine, and the arms are usually tucked to the sides with a shoulder roll in place.

133. C: A minor instrument tray would be the most helpful tray on the list for repair of an inguinal hernia, direct or indirect.

134. A: A pancreaticoduodenectomy, or Whipple procedure, is often performed when the patient has widespread malignancy or severe pancreatitis. In this procedure, the head of the pancreas, duodenum, as well as a portion of the jejunum, stomach, and common bile duct are removed.

135. B: Laparoscopic Nissen fundoplication surgeries are used to treat gastroesophageal reflux disease (GERD) and hiatal hernias.

136. B: A pyloroplasty enlarges the gastric outlet to increase stomach emptying. This procedure is often performed in conjunction with a vagotomy.

137. C: ESWL, also known as extracorporeal shock wave lithotripsy, is a procedure that uses shock waves to break up kidney stones so the patient may excrete them safely.

138. B: During a decortication of a lung, the restrictive tissue is stripped away from the pleura to enhance respiration.

139. B: A thymectomy is usually performed through a sternal splitting incision.

140. C: In order to continue cerebral perfusion when the carotid vessels are clamped, a commercially prepared tube known as a shunt device is often used. A Javid shunt is an example of such a device.

141. B: Lasers of any kind can be a safety hazard and should always be placed in "standby" mode when not in use. Usually, the equipment tech will do this automatically, but the surgical team members should also be aware to avoid injury.

142. A: Many sharps, such as hypodermic needles and suture needles, are not recommended for reprocessing. In addition, suture material itself can have decreased strength if reprocessed. The other three items are commonly reprocessed.

143. B: Endoscopic light sources can become very hot and may start a fire when left on surgical drapes unattended. Whenever a light is not in use, it should be placed on standby mode to prevent risk of burn injury and fire.

144. B: It is important to perform a leak test before the scope is submerged to ensure the seals are in good working condition; otherwise, fluids can get into the head of the scope and damage it.

145. C: A Maryland dissector forceps is an endoscopic instrument most commonly used in laparoscopic procedures. In this case, the laparoscopic cholecystectomy is the only option in which this instrument would be used.

146. A: A cystotomy is an opening made into the bladder, and a drainage tube, usually a Foley or Malecot catheter, is entered into it.

147. B: The Marshall–Marchetti procedure, also known as a vesicourethral suspension, is used for stress urinary incontinence.

148. C: A Litvak Pereyra needle is a ligature needle used in bladder neck suspensions to help pull the sutures of the suspension mesh upward and secure them.

149. D: The United Network of Organ Sharing (UNOS) identifies each organ for transplant with a special number known as the UNOS number.

150. C: University of Wisconsin (UW) solution, or ViaSpan, is a medication used as an organ flush after harvesting in preparation for transplant. Of the choices listed, a living donor nephrectomy would be the only correct choice.

151. D: The first to sixth months have the highest risk for infections because the immunosuppression therapy is still at a high dose, putting the patient at risk for all types of infections.

152. B: There are four quadrants to the Perioperative Patient Focused Model. Three are patient focused, and one is related to the healthcare facility the care is provided.

153. C: It is recommended that surgical attire be low linting to prevent foreign bodies' entrance into the sterile area. It should be changed daily, even if it has not become soiled. Although disposable scrubs are acceptable, reusable ones can also be used as long as they meet the proper requirements.

154. B: Wearing surgical attire helps prevent bacterial shedding from the human body, in the form of hair, dead skin, and other particles. It also helps control the surgical environment by eliminating items from outside that might be on a perioperative personnel's clothing that could cause a surgical site infection, such as pet hair.

155. C: As long as the fluid is not expired, you can keep it after it is removed from the warming cabinet but you cannot rewarm it. It is recommended that you place a "Do Not Rewarm" label on the bottle and store it at room temperature until the manufacturer's recommended expiration date.

156. C: Although the surgeon might suggest it, you should never warm irrigation or IV fluids by placing them in the microwave or a warm autoclave. Because there is no temperature control with these methods, the patient and team members could sustain burn injuries with this method. The most effective way to safely heat fluids is through the use of a specially designed fluid warming cabinet or a portable fluid warmer. These items are set at the recommended range and have a digital readout so you may verify the safe temperature of the fluids before use on the patient.

157. D: Dextran is a nonelectrolyte fluid that is safe with monopolar electrosurgery, but it is a derivative of beet sugar and should not be used on persons with this allergy, allergy to the fluid media itself, or hemostatic illnesses. It is not recommended to use more than 500 mL of this solution during the surgery.

158. C: Sorbitol is routinely used as a urologic irrigation.

159. C: Although keeping track of fluids in and out will help with the determination of blood loss, the most important reason is to determine if a fluid deficit is occurring. In this particular surgery, the patient can absorb fluid media into the vascular system, which can cause many complications, and even death.

160. C: The internal ties are the only ones that are not in contact with the exterior sterile portion of the gown; therefore, they are the only ones the circulator or other nonsterile team members may touch to help gown the surgeon.

161. D: The external waist tie attached by a tag must be passed to the circulating nurse so the gown can finish being tied and closed. The back of the gown cannot be open. The circulating nurse holds the tag at the designated area, while the surgeon turns. He then takes the sterile tie out of the tag, without touching the portion the circulator has.

162. B: The sterile external tie can be placed inside a sterile glove wrapper to prevent contamination when the circulator takes it to help the surgeon turn and finish tying the surgical gown.

163. A: Compressed air and nitrogen are the only two gas sources that should be used with a pneumatic tourniquet. Nitrous oxide and oxygen should never be used because they increase the risk of fire.

164. B: Any facility that procures and/or stores human tissue must register with the FDA as a tissue bank. If the facility just purchases tissue for use in that facility or stores tissue for use on the same patient, this is not necessary.

165. A: Tissue storage freezers and refrigerators should be checked a minimum of once a day to ensure they are within the proper temperature range for the tissue stored.

166. D: Sponge counts should be done before the case, at the closure of each cavity, before the wound is closed, after the wound is closed, and upon any permanent relief of staff.

167. D: All the other items are detectable on a radiograph except nonradiopaque towels. For this reason, they should never be used in a wound due to the risk of retention.

168. C: Any surgery where the team sees a risk for a retained instrument, instrument counts should be performed. These counts are done at the same frequency as sponge and sharp counts.

169. A: Personnel who must remain close to the surgical field, such as the scrubbed team members, should wear thyroid shields and leaded glasses because these areas are very sensitive to radiation exposure.

170. D: In this situation, only the radiology tech should be moving the C-arm. Only trained personnel with proper state licensing should operate these devices.

171. A: Surgical specimens should be specially handled and listed as either surgical pathology examination (routine), gross examination, or disposal. Frozen section and permanent are examples of surgical pathology.

172. D: It is very important to carefully handle and document forensic specimens from the time of removal from the patient to examination. This information establishes the chain of custody of this evidence. This is particularly important if the specimen is involved in a criminal investigation.

173. C: By pulling up the sleeves of the gown, it allows the surgeon's fingers and hand to pass into the awaiting sterile glove easier. The other answers may cause the scrub nurse to contaminate her sterile gloves.

174. B: Bariatric surgery includes procedures such as gastric banding and gastric bypass, which is predominately performed for weight loss.

175. C: Among many others, gastroesophageal reflux disease, also known as GERD, is an associated disease with morbid obesity. This is significant to surgical procedures because the patient's gag reflex is unprotected when given anesthesia and the patient may aspirate. Providing cricoid pressure during induction is often requested for this purpose.

176. C: Roux-en-Y gastric bypass is the only procedure listed that is a combination of the two bariatric surgery approaches: restrictive and malabsorptive. Both proximal gastric bypass and banding are restrictive, and jejunoileal bypass is a malabsorptive.

177. C: Adjustable gastric bands to have a possible complication of tissue erosion if the band slips. The other complications are specific to gastric bypass procedures.

178. B: These patients are placed in the reverse Trendelenburg position, and placement of a padded footboard helps to prevent slipping down the table and causing patient injury.

179. D: Laryngeal nerve paralysis is a possible complication when administering a brachial plexus nerve block.

180. A: A scleral buckling procedure is performed for retinal detachment.

181. B: Labyrinthectomy is performed for severe vertigo. A stapedectomy is performed for some hearing loss diseases. Pressure equalization (PE) tubes would be more helpful in patients with chronic ear infections. Mastoidectomy is used to treat cholesteatoma.

182. B: The Alvarado foot holder is a type of positioning equipment that keeps the patient's leg bent to provide stability and visualization during total knee arthroplasty procedures.

183. C: There are three types of dermatomes, and they are used for removing tissue that will be used in skin grafting.

184. B: Loupes are magnifying eyeglasses that the surgeon wears during microsurgery, in this case to see the small sutures used in the procedure.

185. A: The draping materials form a barrier and must be fluid resistant and resistant to tearing or puncture to avoid microbial penetration. A sterile drape should be lint free to reduce airborne contaminates and shedding onto the surgical site.

186. A: A special consideration for correct draping is to ensure that the prep solutions have dried before applying surgical drapes. Pooled prep fluids can cause skin breakdown. These fluids, especially those containing alcohol, can also be flammable when still in liquid form.

187. A: Shifting of the drapes can cause bacteria from nonprepped skin to be dragged into the sterile field. Also, the more the drape is moved, the higher the chances that it will come into contact with surrounding nonsterile furniture or fall below the sterile field.

188. C: Draping should begin at the surgical site and move to the periphery to reduce contamination from nonprepped skin areas.

189. C: To prevent injury, sharps should be passed in a "hands-free" manner in a safe zone, such as placing the knife handle in an emesis basin.

190. B: Keeping the doors closed helps to reduce the number of microbes in the OR suite. This is true whether a surgery is occurring or not.

191. B: One of the risks of a carotid endarterectomy is possible damage to the nerves that control the movement of the vocal cords. Paralysis of the vocal cords can cause many complications, including difficulty breathing.

192. A: It is important for a "time out" to be called before any procedure, including regional anesthetic procedures. The patient should have been identified at the preoperative level and with the anesthesia care provider when first brought into the OR suite.

193. A: Air embolism is a potential complication of intercostal nerve blocks.

194. C: A and B refer to spinal and epidural anesthesia. Digits are one of the many possible injection sites for nerve blocks.

195. A: Introducing a nerve block dose of local medication into the bloodstream can lead to toxicity and a possible cardiac arrest. This can happen during a Bier block if the tourniquet is deflated too quickly.

196. A: The patient's name and date of birth are two pieces of information that can be properly used to identify the patient.

197. D: Arteriovenous fistula patients are at risk for hemorrhage at the fistula site. This risk does not dissipate after surgery. These patients are at risk for a life-threatening hemorrhage even years after the procedure if the fistula develops an aneurysm.

198. A: Although all of these forms contain important information, the patient's consent is the only one of the four reviewed for verification of the procedure.

199. A: All team members should verbalize agreement with the proposed information in the "time out."

200. D: One of the many things that should be checked during the head-to-toe assessment is the neurovascular area. Assessing peripheral pulses is one method to do this.

Made in the USA
Middletown, DE
22 February 2018